CONTENTS

CHAPTER 4 FISH AND SEAFOOD......38

CHAPTER 5 POULTRY......50

CHAPTER 6 BEEF 65

CHAPTER 7 PORK 77

CHAPTER 15 DESSERTS..134

RECIPE INDEX...143

INTRODUCTION

The success of Instant Pot seems to be everywhere in the world. In recent years, an army of these programmable pressure cookers has appeared on kitchen counters around the world. Instant Pots seems to have attracted the hearts of countless home cooks overnight.

The uniqueness and advantages of Instant Pot attracted me when Instant Pot coming to the market. I bought my first Instant Pot two years ago. After receiving the Instant Pot, I could not wait to open the box and use it for cooking. At first, I cooked many different dishes according to the bonus recipes manual. It didn't take long for me to cook all the recipes. So, I started searching for relevant Instant Pot recipes from the Internet, and recorded those delicious and easy-to-use dishes one by one in my own blank recipe book. At the same time, I was not satisfied with the first Instant Pot I bought. Later I bought two Instant Pot of different models and sizes to facilitate the use of different occasions. Two years have passed, and I have accumulated a large number of delicious and simple Instant Pot recipes, including simple breakfast, chicken soup, porridge, delicious slow-cooked beef brisket, desserts and more.

With the popularity of Instant Pot, the demand for Instant Pot recipes from home cooks is also increasing. Therefore, I would like to share some of my experience and over 1000 accumulated recipes in the past two years with readers. I hope that this book becomes a new classic in your kitchen and encourages you to plug in your Instant Pot and get cooking right away. If you're new to Instant Pot cooking, welcome! I will tell you the everything about Instant Pot to you in the Chapter 1.

CHAPTER 1 UNDERSTANDING THE INSTANT POT

Whether you have already bought it or you are thinking about buying an instant pot, know that this revolutionary appliance will be the star of your kitchen and your new best friend. Why? Because it replaces 7 different kitchen gadgets. That being said, you can use your one and not-expensive Instant Pot for 7 different cooking methods:

1. A Pressure Cooker
2. A Sauté Pan
3. A Slow Cooker
4. A Steamer
5. A Rice Cooker
6. A Yogurt Maker
7. A Warming Pot

Why Choose the Instant Pot?

If you're still in two minds about the advantages of owning a multicooker, here are some further reasons why an Instant Pot is one of the top kitchen appliances out there.

Easy and Effortless
There's no need to check on the food, as it's continuously cooked. You don't have to constantly stir or keep an eye on the temperature to make sure nothing burns. The only effort you have to go through is prepping the vegetables and meat and putting it all in the pot! In a few minutes, you'll have a warm meal to share with your family.

Safe and Secure
You can relax knowing that there's no possibility that your Instant Pot will blow up. This modern-day cooker has built-in safety features and sensors that the old-school pressure cookers don't have.

Straightforward to Clean
One would think that an appliance with the ability to cook a whole meal will require some aftercare hassles and complicated cleaning instructions. Not at all! There's only one inner pot and a few smaller elements to wash, and they're all dishwasher safe. Gone are the days of having to wash three pots, casseroles, and utensils galore.

No Nutrients Go to Waste
It's an unfortunate fact that the longer you cook food, the more nutrients go to waste. But, seeing that the cooking time is so much shorter when you use a multicooker, your food will still be loaded with vitamins and minerals.

Gets Rid of Germs
Your kitchen may be spotless, but there's no way of knowing if the food you're bringing from outside is bacteria-free. Luckily, since the Instant Pot not only cooks food at a low temperature but also under pressure, bacteria and germs will die during the process.

No Shortage of Recipes
Not only will you find recipes in this book, but you can also do a quick internet search and be flooded with Instant Pot recipe blogs. You'll find anything from making a delicious beef stew, to how to make yogurt, and even wine!

It's exciting, right? Now that you know what makes the Instant Pot special, it is time to look at factors you should keep in mind when selecting your multicooker.

What to Do When You Get Your Cooker?

You will see the following when you open the box your cooker came in (apart from the actual Instant Pot, of course):

Manual

Quick reference guide

Condensation collector

Steamer rack

Soup scoop

Rice measuring cup

Rice paddle

Recipe book

The manual and quick reference guide will give you all the information required to set up your cooker. Read through it properly. While some multicookers will come already assembled, others do not, and you will have to install the inner pot, sealing ring, and the lid.

Before you do, wash all the elements with warm water and dry with a cloth. Wipe—do not submerge—the Instant Pot with a warm wet cloth and then dry. When all elements are completely dry, you can insert the inner pot. Next, put in the sealing ring and make sure it is fixed securely. Make sure all other components of the lid are in place by referring to the manual.

Once done, you're ready to test your pot!

Water Test

Although it is not absolutely necessary to do this step, I recommend you do it, nonetheless. It will give you peace of mind that the Instant Pot is in complete working order.

After assembling your multicooker and reading through the manual and quick reference guide to see what all the buttons do and icons mean, it is time to go through a water test.

1. Plug the cooker into the wall socket and switch it on.
2. Place the inner pot inside the cooker and add three cups of water.
3. Make sure the sealing ring is inserted securely.
4. Seal the Instant Pot with the lid. You will hear the pot beep three times to indicate that the lid is sealed.
5. Select 'Sealing' on the steam release handle.
6. Press the Pressure Cook/Steam button and set the timer to two minutes. Then press 'Start.'
7. If a lot of steam is escaping out of the sides, switch the machine off, and check the silicone ring is in place correctly. Try again.
8. Once the pot comes to pressure, a countdown will begin. The water should be boiling after two minutes. If that is the case, your water test was successful, and your Instant Pot doesn't have any defects.

How Does It Work?

I know it can be overwhelming when you first get your Instant Pot. Don't worry, after reading this section you'll be ready to dish up your first culinary masterpiece!

So, first things first: How does it actually work?

The cooker is made up out of three components called the inner pot, the cooker base, and the lid.

The **inner pot** is the container that goes inside the actual cooker. You will put all your ingredients in this part of the cooker. As the liquid inside the inner pot heats, it creates steam that cannot escape. This, in turn, creates pressure.

The **cooker base** is where all the electric and safety mechanisms are housed. The microprocessor, pressure and temperature sensors, heating element, and display and control panel all form part of this element.

The **lid** is a critical part of your multicooker; if it doesn't seal completely, the pot will not come to pressure. The lid itself contains numerous small parts, including the steam release, sealing ring, float valve and silicone cap, and anti-block shield. All of these work together to seal and regulate pressure.

The **steam release** can be set to either venting or sealed, and also acts as a safety feature where if the pressure increases to an unsafe level, the excess steam will push the valve up to release pressure.

The **sealing ring** is made from durable silicone rubber and creates an airtight seal.

The **float valve and silicone cap** fully seal the cooker. The float valve also acts as a latch lock, which prevents the lid from turning when force is applied.

The **anti-block shield** prevents blockage of the steam release pipe and ensures a steady release of steam when depressurizing.

Okay, now that you know what each of the components does, let's have a look at the buttons and icons.

The Buttons

The exact buttons will depend on the model and make you have, so you will have to use the user manual as guidance when you're unsure. But I will cover the general buttons for your convenience.

Sauté

You can use this multicooker to sauté food as you would using a skillet. The Instant Pot will warm to the temperature you selected (low, normal/medium, high) and let you know with a beep that you can start sautéing.

The time limit for this specific setting is 30-minutes, but you will usually only need 10 to 15 minutes. If you do require more time, just press the 'Sauté' button again, and you'll have 30 more minutes.

Be sure to add a little oil to ensure food doesn't get stuck to the bottom of the pan.

Manual or Pressure Cook

Your machine will either have a 'Manual' or 'Pressure cook' button. This is what you'll press if you want your pot to come to pressure.

Setting the Cooking Time

You have to let your pot know for how long it must cook. Just hit the plus or minus button to set the amount of time required per the recipe you're following. It will take a few seconds for 'On' to display, and your pot will start to build pressure. On some models, the timer is set by turning a knob and hitting 'Start.' Usually, on these models, the timer countdown will only begin once the cooker has come to pressure, and the cooking process has started.

When the time is up, you will see L0:00 or 00:00 appear on the screen. The timer will then start counting up to indicate how long it has been since the cooking process concluded. This is essential information when a recipe calls for a timed natural release (more on that later).

Keep Warm/Cancel

Your cooker may have these buttons separately or as one. For the "Keep Warm" function, most Instant Pots will automatically revert to this setting when the cooking time has ended.

If you want to cancel a function or switch to another, press the 'Cancel' button. This is also the button you will use to turn off your Instant Pot after use. Just hold in the 'Cancel' button for a few seconds until 'Off' is displayed on the screen.

Delay Start

A delayed start is convenient if you want cooking to start later on. I use this function almost every day. You can prep the ingredients, add them to the pot, and then set the timer so that the food is ready when your guests arrive. Just think, no more running between the kitchen while entertaining friends or family—the multicooker does everything for you.

Just keep in mind that not all food is safe to stay out of the refrigerator for too long before cooking. Chicken is a good example of meat you won't be able to place in the pot in the morning to start cooking four to six hours later.

Pressure/Steam Release

The lid is an important aspect when it comes to the pressure/steam release of your Instant Pot. Although the lids of various models differ slightly, they all have two positions: venting and sealing.

You will position the pressure release on 'Sealing' when you want to pressure cook anything. When the cooking process is done, you will move the position to 'Venting' to allow steam to escape and depressurizing to take place.

There, however, are three different types of pressure release methods. If you're following a specific recipe, this information will be included. The method you end up using also depends on the type of food in the pot.

Quick pressure release (QPR) is when you let all the steam escape at once. Foods like fish, veggies, or anything else that doesn't require a lot of cooking time will make use of QPR.

Natural pressure release (NPR) is when you don't move the pressure release to venting at all but instead let the pot depressurize as it cools. This can take anywhere from a few minutes up to 10 hours. The "Keep Warm" function automatically kicks in once cooking has stopped, the pot will stay on for 10 hours during which it will slowly depressurize.

Timed NPR is where you wait a certain amount of time before venting the steam. The recipe you're using will usually indicate how long you should wait.

The Icons

If you buy a basic multicooker, it will come with a red or blue LED. The more expensive models have digital screens, and you will see different icons appear at certain times during the process.

Flame under a pot

The pot is busy warming up. The icon will also go on and off as the pot regulates its heat while cooking.

'P' in a pot

The "Pressure Cook" function is selected.

Thermometer

"Keep Warm" mode has been activated.

Speaker with an 'X' next to it

All sounds have been muted. If your pot still makes sound and you would like to turn it off, do the following:

On the Duo, Duo Plus, Duo Nova, SV, or Viva models, press the minus button until the machine displays 'Off.' Alternatively, to turn it on, you will have to press the plus button until 'On' is shown.

If you own an Ultra or Duo Evo Plus, while 'Off' is displayed on the screen, press and hold the knob for a few seconds. You can then turn the knob to select 'On' or 'Off,' and press the knob again to set the sound setting in place.

The Best Cooker for You

There are various makes and models on the market, and this makes it hard to know which one will fulfill your needs. Ask yourself the questions below, and you'll be able to get the right multicooker for you.

How big is your family?

If you're only cooking for two, then there's no need to buy an 8-quart cooker. Here are the breakdowns of the different sizes.

3-quart = one or two people

6-quart = three to six people

8-quart = six to nine people

8 Safety Cooking Tips

Furthermore, there are some safety tips you need to keep in mind:

Check that the inner pot and heating plate are both clean and dry.

Check the lid for any stuck food particles. Pay extra attention to the float valve, exhaust valve, and anti-block shield.

Check the sealing ring is secure.

Check the steam release valve is set to 'Sealing.'

Make sure not to overfill the Instant Pot. At no time should the contents in the pot surpass the three-quarter mark. If you're cooking starchy foods, the halfway mark is ideal.

Be careful when you release the steam.

Unplug the multicooker when not in use.

No part of the pot that contains electrical components should be submerged in water.

Pressure Release

It may seem complicated to pressure cook your meals, but the Instant Pot is the most hassle-free appliance among its fellow pressure cookers. There are two ways in which you can release the pressure:

Quick Pressure Release (QPR) – If you choose this method, you will let the pressure out of the pot quickly and all at once. You can use this with seafood, veggies, or even meat. Just make sure that your pot isn't full because it will result in spillage.

Naturally Pressure Release (NPR) – When the food you are cooking is larger in volute, is foamy, or has a high liquid content, a natural pressure release is required in order to prevent leaking.

Timed Natural Pressure Release - I often wait 10 or 15 minutes after the end of a cooking program, then move the Pressure Release to Venting to release a less geyser-like amount of steam from the pot.

Cooking Time Chart

Now is the time when you'll realize just how much time an Instant Pot will save you in the kitchen!

Food	Cooking Time
Vegetables	
Asparagus	1-2 min
Broccoli	1-2 min
Brussel sprouts	2-3 min
Cabbage (whole)	2-3 min
Beans	1-2 min
Butternut squash	4-6 min
Carrots	6-8 min
Corn on the cob	3-5 min
Potatoes (Large)	12-15 min
Potatoes (Small)	8-10 min
Potatoes (Cubes)	3-5 min
Sweet potatoes (Whole)	12-15 min
Sweet potatoes (Cubes)	2-4 min
Cauliflower (florets)	2-3 min
Mixed vegetables	3-4 min
Meat, Fish, & Eggs	
Beef stew	20 min (per 1lb)
Beef large	20-25 min (per 1lb)
Beef ribs	20-25 min (per 1lb)
Chicken whole	8 min (per 1lb)

Chicken breasts	6-8 min (per 1lb)
Chicken bone stock	40-45 min (per 1lb)
Lamb leg	15 min (per 1lb)
Pork roast	15 min (per 1lb)
Pork baby back ribs	15-20 min (per 1lb)
Fish whole	4-5 min
Fish fillet	2-3 min
Lobster	2-3 min
Shrimp	1-3 min
Seafood stock	7-8 min
Eggs	5 min
Rice & Grains	
Barley	20-22 min
Oatmeal	2-3 min
Oats	3-5 min
Quinoa	1 min
Porridge	5-7 min
Rice (Brown)	20-22 min
Rice (Jasmine)	4 min
Rice (Basmati)	2-3 min
Rice (White)	4 min
Rice (Wild)	20-25 min
Beans & Lentils (Dry)	

Black Beans	20-25 min
Kidney Beans (Red)	20-25 min
Kidney Beans (White)	25-30 min
Lima Beans	12-14 min
Lentils (Green)	8-10 min
Lentils (Yellow)	1-2 min
Chickpeas	30-40 min
Navy Beans	20-24 min
Pinto Beans	25-30 min
Soy Beans	35-45 min

CHAPTER 2 BREAKFAST AND BRUNCH

Bacon and Egg Risotto

Prep time: 12 mins, Cook Time: 12 mins, Servings: 2

- 1½ cups chicken stock
- 2 poached eggs
- 2 tbsps. grated Parmesan cheese
- 3 chopped bacon slices
- ¾ cup Arborio rice

1. Set your Instant Pot to Sauté and add the bacon and cook for 5 minutes until crispy, stirring occasionally.
2. Carefully stir in the rice and let cook for an additional 1 minute.
3. Add the chicken stock and stir well.
4. Lock the lid. Select the Manual mode and set the cooking time for 6 minutes at Low Pressure.
5. Once cooking is complete, do a quick pressure release. Carefully open the lid.
6. Add the Parmesan cheese and keep stirring until melted. Divide the risotto between two plates. Add the eggs on the side and serve immediately.

Eggs En Cocotte

Prep time: 10 mins, Cook Time: 20 mins, Servings: 4

- 1 cup water
- 1 tbsp. butter
- 4 tbsps. heavy whipping cream
- 4 eggs
- 1 tbsp. chives
- Salt and pepper, to taste

1. Arrange a steamer rack in the Instant Pot, then pour in the water.
2. Grease four ramekins with butter.
3. Divide the heavy whipping cream in the ramekins, then break each egg in each ramekin.
4. Sprinkle them with chives, salt, and pepper.
5. Arrange the ramekins on the steamer rack.
6. Lock the lid. Set to the Manual mode, then set the timer for 20 minutes at High Pressure.
7. Once the timer goes off, perform a natural pressure release for 10 minutes, then release any remaining pressure. Carefully open the lid.

8. Transfer them on a plate and serve immediately.

Eggs In Purgatory

Prep time: 15 minutes | Cook time: 24 minutes | Serves 4

2 (14½-ounce / 411-g) cans fire-roasted diced tomatoes, undrained
½ cup water
1 medium onion, chopped
2 garlic cloves, minced
2 tablespoons canola oil
2 teaspoons smoked paprika
½ teaspoon crushed red pepper flakes
½ teaspoon sugar
¼ cup tomato paste
4 large eggs
¼ cup shredded Monterey Jack cheese
2 tablespoons minced fresh parsley
1 (18-ounce / 510-g) tube polenta, sliced and warmed (optional)

1. Place the tomatoes, water, onion, garlic, oil, paprika, red pepper flakes, and sugar into the Instant Pot and stir to combine.
2. Secure the lid. Select the Manual mode and set the cooking time for 4 minutes at High Pressure.
3. Once cooking is complete, do a quick pressure release. Carefully open the lid.
4. Set the Instant Pot to Sauté and stir in the tomato paste. Let it simmer for about 10 minutes, stirring occasionally, or until the mixture is slightly thickened.
5. With the back of a spoon, make 4 wells in the sauce and crack an egg into each. Scatter with the shredded cheese.
6. Cover (do not lock the lid) and allow to simmer for 8 to 10 minutes, or until the egg whites are completely set.
7. Sprinkle the parsley on top and serve with the polenta slices, if desired.

Vanilla Pancake

Prep time: 5 minutes | Cook time: 50 minutes | Serves 6

3 eggs, beaten
½ cup coconut flour
¼ cup heavy cream
¼ cup almond flour
3 tablespoons Swerve
1 teaspoon vanilla extract
1 teaspoon baking powder
Cooking spray

1. In a bowl, stir together the eggs, coconut flour, heavy cream, almond flour, Swerve and vanilla extract. Whisk in the baking powder until smooth.
2. Spritz the bottom and sides of Instant Pot with cooking spray. Place the batter in the pot.
3. Set the lid in place. Select the Manual mode and set the cooking time for 50 minutes on Low Pressure. Once the timer goes off, perform a natural pressure release for 5 minutes, then release any remaining pressure. Carefully open the lid.
4. Let the pancake rest in the pot for 5 minutes before serving.

French Eggs

Prep time: 12 mins, Cook Time: 8 mins, Servings: 4

- ¼ tsp. salt
- 4 bacon slices
- 1 tbsp. olive oil
- 4 tbsps. chopped chives
- 4 eggs
- 1½ cups water

1. Grease 4 ramekins with a drizzle of oil and crack an egg into each ramekin.
2. Add a bacon slice on top and season with salt. Sprinkle the chives on top.
3. Add 1½ cups water and steamer basket to your Instant Pot. Transfer the ramekins to the basket.
4. Lock the lid. Select the Manual mode and set the cooking time for 8 minutes at High Pressure.
5. Once cooking is complete, do a quick pressure release. Carefully open the lid.

6. Serve your baked eggs immediately.

Asparagus and Gruyère Cheese Frittata

Prep time: 10 minutes | Cook time: 22 minutes | Serves 6

6 eggs
6 tablespoons heavy cream
½ teaspoon salt
½ teaspoon black pepper
1 tablespoon butter
2½ ounces (71 g) asparagus, chopped
1 clove garlic, minced
1¼ cup shredded Gruyère cheese, divided
Cooking spray
3 ounces (85 g) halved cherry tomatoes
½ cup water

1. In a large bowl, stir together the eggs, cream, salt, and pepper.
2. Set the Instant Pot on the Sauté mode and melt the butter. Add the asparagus and garlic to the pot and sauté for 2 minutes, or until the garlic is fragrant. The asparagus should still be crisp.
3. Transfer the asparagus and garlic to the bowl with the egg mixture. Stir in 1 cup of the cheese. Clean the pot.
4. Spritz a baking pan with cooking spray. Spread the tomatoes in a single layer in the pan. Pour the egg mixture on top of the tomatoes and sprinkle with the remaining ¼ cup of the cheese. Cover the pan tightly with aluminum foil.
5. Pour the water in the Instant Pot and insert the trivet. Place the pan on the trivet.
6. Set the lid in place. Select the Manual mode and set the cooking time for 20 minutes on High Pressure. When the timer goes off, perform a quick pressure release. Carefully open the lid.
7. Remove the pan from the pot and remove the foil. Blot off any excess moisture with a paper towel. Let the frittata cool for 5 to 10 minutes before transferring onto a plate.

Spinach and Ham Frittata

Prep time: 3 mins, Cook Time: 10 mins, Servings: 8
- 1 cup diced ham
- 2 cups chopped spinach
- 8 eggs, beaten
- ½ cup coconut milk
- 1 onion, chopped
- 1 tsp. salt

1. Put all the ingredients into the Instant Pot. Stir to mix well.
2. Lock the lid. Set to Manual mode, then set the timer for 10 minutes at High Pressure.
3. Once the timer goes off, perform a natural pressure release for 5 minutes. Carefully open the lid.
4. Transfer the frittata on a plate and serve immediately.

Hawaiian Sweet Potato Hash

Prep time: 20 minutes | Cook time: 20 minutes | Serves 6
4 bacon strips, chopped
1 tablespoon canola or coconut oil
2 large sweet potatoes, peeled and cut into ½-inch pieces
1 cup water
2 cups cubed fresh pineapple
½ teaspoon salt
¼ teaspoon paprika
¼ teaspoon chili powder
¼ teaspoon pepper
⅛ teaspoon ground cinnamon
1. Press the Sauté button on the Instant Pot and add the bacon. Cook for about 7 minutes, stirring occasionally, or until crisp.
2. Remove the bacon with a slotted spoon and drain on paper towels. Set aside.
3. In the Instant Pot, heat the oil until it shimmers.
4. Working in batches, add the sweet potatoes to the pot and brown each side for 3 to 4 minutes. Transfer the sweet potatoes to a large bowl and set aside.
5. Pour the water into the pot and cook for 1 minute, stirring to loosen browned bits from pan.
6. Place a steamer basket in the Instant Pot. Add the pineapple, salt, paprika, chili powder, pepper, and cinnamon to the large bowl of sweet potatoes and toss well, then transfer the mixture to the steamer basket.
7. Secure the lid. Select the Steam mode and set the cooking time for 2 minutes at High Pressure.
8. Once cooking is complete, do a quick pressure release. Carefully open the lid.
9. Top with the bacon and serve on a plate.

Buttery Herbed Sirloin Steak

Prep time: 5 minutes | Cook time: 1 minute | Serves 2
½ cup water
1 pound (454 g) boneless beef sirloin steak
½ teaspoon salt
½ teaspoon black pepper
1 clove garlic, minced
2 tablespoons butter, softened
¼ teaspoon dried rosemary
¼ teaspoon dried parsley
Pinch of dried thyme
1. Pour the water into the Instant Pot and put the trivet in the pot.
2. Rub the steak all over with salt and black pepper. Place the steak on the trivet.
3. In a small bowl, stir together the remaining ingredients. Spread half of the butter mixture over the steak.
4. Set the lid in place. Select the Manual mode and set the cooking time for 1 minute on Low Pressure. When the timer goes off, perform a quick pressure release. Carefully open the lid.
5. Remove the steak from the pot. Top with the remaining half of the butter mixture. Serve hot.

Cheese and Spinach Strata

Prep time: 5 minutes | Cook time: 40 minutes | Serves 4
1 cup filtered water
6 eggs
1 cup chopped spinach
1 cup shredded full-fat Cheddar cheese
¼ small onion, thinly sliced

½ tablespoon salted grass-fed butter, softened

½ teaspoon Dijon mustard

½ teaspoon kosher salt

½ teaspoon freshly ground black pepper

½ teaspoon cayenne pepper

½ teaspoon paprika

½ teaspoon dried sage

½ teaspoon dried cilantro

½ teaspoon dried parsley

1.   Pour the water into the the Instant Pot, then place the trivet.

2.   Whisk together the eggs, spinach, cheese, onion, butter, mustard, salt, black pepper, cayenne pepper, paprika, sage, cilantro, and parsley in a large bowl until well incorporated. Pour the egg mixture into a greased baking dish. Cover the dish loosely with aluminum foil. Put the dish on top of the trivet.

3.   Secure the lid. Select the Manual mode and set the cooking time for 40 minutes at High Pressure.

4.   Once cooking is complete, do a natural pressure release for 10 minutes, then release any remaining pressure. Carefully open the lid.

5.   Let the strata rest for 5 minutes and serve warm.

Cabbage and Zucchini Hash Browns

Prep time: 5 minutes | Cook time: 8 minutes | Serves 3

1 cup shredded white cabbage

3 eggs, beaten

½ teaspoon ground nutmeg

½ teaspoon salt

½ teaspoon onion powder

½ zucchini, grated

1 tablespoon coconut oil

1.   In a bowl, stir together all the ingredients, except for the coconut oil. Form the cabbage mixture into medium hash browns.

2.   Press the Sauté button on the Instant Pot and heat the coconut oil.

3.   Place the hash browns in the hot coconut oil. Cook for 4 minutes on each side, or until lightly browned.

4.   Transfer the hash browns to a plate and serve warm.

Lettuce Wrapped Chicken Sandwich

Prep time: 10 minutes | Cook time: 15 minutes | Serves 4

1 tablespoon butter

3 ounces (85 g) scallions, chopped

2 cups ground chicken

½ teaspoon ground nutmeg

1 tablespoon coconut flour

1 teaspoon salt

1 cup lettuce

1.   Press the Sauté button on the Instant Pot and melt the butter. Add the chopped scallions, ground chicken and ground nutmeg to the pot and sauté for 4 minutes. Add the coconut flour and salt and continue to sauté for 10 minutes.

2.   Fill the lettuce with the ground chicken and transfer it on the plate. Serve immediately.

Buckwheat Breakfast Bowls

Prep time: 5 minutes | Cook time: 1 minute | Serves 6

2 cups buckwheat groats, soaked for at least 20 minutes and up to overnight

3 cups water

¼ cup pure maple syrup

1 teaspoon vanilla extract

1 teaspoon ground cinnamon

¼ teaspoon fine sea salt

Almond milk, for serving

Chopped or sliced fresh fruit, for serving

1.   Drain and rinse the buckwheat. In the Instant Pot, combine the buckwheat with the water, maple syrup, cinnamon, vanilla, and salt.

2.   Lock the lid. Select the Manual mode and set the cooking time for 1 minute at High Pressure.

3.   When the timer beeps, perform a natural pressure release for 10 minutes, then release any remaining pressure. Carefully remove the lid and stir the cooked grains.

4.   Serve the buckwheat warm with almond milk and fresh fruit.

Steel-Cut Oatmeal

Prep time: 5 minutes | Cook time: 14 minutes | Serves 2

½ cup steel-cut oats

1½ cups water

¼ cup maple syrup, plus additional as needed

2 tablespoons packed brown sugar

¼ teaspoon ground cinnamon

Pinch kosher salt, plus additional as needed

1 tablespoon unsalted butter

1. Press the Sauté button on the Instant Pot. Add the steel-cut oats and toast for about 2 minutes, stirring occasionally.

2. Add the water, ¼ cup of maple syrup, brown sugar, cinnamon, and pinch salt to the Instant Pot and stir well.

3. Lock the lid. Select the Manual mode and set the cooking time for 12 minutes at High Pressure.

4. Once cooking is complete, do a natural pressure release for 10 minutes, then release any remaining pressure. Carefully open the lid.

5. Stir the oatmeal and taste, adding additional maple syrup or salt as needed.

6. Let the oatmeal sit for 10 minutes. When ready, add the butter and stir well. Ladle into bowls and serve immediately.

Mini Bell Pepper and Cheddar Frittata

Prep time: 12 mins, Cook Time: 5 mins, Servings: 6

- 1 chopped red bell pepper
- 1 tbsp. almond milk
- ¼ tsp. salt
- 2 tbsps. grated Cheddar cheese
- 5 whisked eggs
- 1½ cups water

1. In a bowl, combine the salt, eggs, cheese, almond milk, and red bell pepper, and whisk well. Pour the egg mixture into 6 baking molds.

2. Add 1½ cups water and steamer basket to your Instant Pot. Transfer the baking molds to the basket.

3. Lock the lid. Select the Manual mode and cook for 5minutes at High Pressure.

4. Once cooking is complete, do a quick pressure release. Carefully open the lid. Serve hot.

Raisin, Apple, and Pecan Oatmeal

Prep time: 10 minutes | Cook time: 5 minutes | Serves 4

¾ cup steel-cut oats

¾ cup raisins

3 cups vanilla almond milk

3 tablespoons brown sugar

4½ teaspoons butter

¾ teaspoon ground cinnamon

½ teaspoon salt

1 large apple, peeled and chopped

¼ cup chopped pecans

1. Combine all the ingredients, except for the apple and pecans, in the Instant Pot.

2. Lock the lid. Select the Manual mode and set the cooking time for 5 minutes at High Pressure.

3. When the timer beeps, perform a natural pressure release for 10 minutes, then release any remaining pressure. Carefully remove the lid.

4. Stir in the apple and let sit for 10 minutes. Spoon the oatmeal into bowls and sprinkle the pecans on top before serving.

Leek and Asparagus Frittata

Prep time: 10 minutes | Cook time: 10 minutes | Serves 4

6 eggs

¼ teaspoon fine sea salt

Freshly ground black pepper, to taste

8 ounces (227 g) asparagus spears, woody stems removed and cut into 1-inch pieces

1 cup thinly sliced leeks

¼ cup grated Parmesan cheese

1 cup water

Chopped green onions, for garnish (optional)

Fresh flat-leaf parsley, for garnish (optional)

1. Whisk together the eggs, salt, and black pepper in a large mixing bowl until frothy.

2. Add the asparagus pieces, leeks, and cheese and stir to combine. Pour the mixture into a greased round cake pan.

3. Add the water and trivet to the Instant Pot, then place the pan on top of the trivet.

4. Lock the lid. Select the Manual mode and set the cooking time for 10 minutes at High Pressure.

5. Once cooking is complete, do a natural pressure release for 10 minutes, then release any remaining pressure. Carefully open the lid.

6. Allow the frittata to cool for 5 minutes. Garnish with the green onions and parsley, if desired. Cut the frittata into wedges and serve warm.

Baked Eggs with Parmesan

Prep time: 5 minutes | Cook time: 10 minutes | Serves 1

1 tablespoon butter, cut into small pieces
2 tablespoons keto-friendly low-carb Marinara sauce
3 eggs
2 tablespoons grated Parmesan cheese
¼ teaspoon Italian seasoning
1 cup water

1. Place the butter pieces on the bottom of the oven-safe bowl. Spread the marinara sauce over the butter. Crack the eggs on top of the marinara sauce and top with the cheese and Italian seasoning.

2. Cover the bowl with aluminum foil. Pour the water and insert the trivet in the Instant Pot. Put the bowl on the trivet.

3. Set the lid in place. Select the Manual mode and set the cooking time for 10 minutes on Low Pressure. When the timer goes off, do a quick pressure release. Carefully open the lid.

4. Let the eggs cool for 5 minutes before serving.

Walnut and Pear Oatmeal

Prep time: 5 minutes | Cook time: 7 minutes | Serves 2

1 cup old-fashioned oats
1¼ cups water
1 medium pear, peeled, cored, and cubed
¼ cup freshly squeezed orange juice
¼ cup chopped walnuts
¼ cup dried cherries
¼ teaspoon ground ginger
¼ teaspoon ground cinnamon
Pinch of salt

1. In the Instant Pot, combine the oats, water, pear, orange juice, walnuts, cherries, ginger, cinnamon, and salt.

2. Secure the lid. Select the Manual mode and set the cooking time for 7 minutes at High Pressure.

3. Once cooking is complete, do a natural pressure release for 10 minutes, then release any remaining pressure. Carefully open the lid.

4. Stir the oatmeal and spoon into two bowls. Serve warm.

Pork Quill Egg Cups

Prep time: 15 minutes | Cook time: 15 minutes | Serves 4

10 ounces (283 g) ground pork
1 jalapeño pepper, chopped
1 tablespoon butter, softened
1 teaspoon dried dill
½ teaspoon salt
1 cup water
4 quill eggs

1. In a bowl, stir together all the ingredients, except for the quill eggs and water. Transfer the meat mixture to the silicone muffin molds and press the surface gently.

2. Pour the water and insert the trivet in the Instant Pot. Put the meat cups on the trivet.

3. Crack the eggs over the meat mixture.

4. Set the lid in place. Select the Manual mode and set the cooking time for 15 minutes on High Pressure. When the timer goes off, do a quick pressure release. Carefully open the lid.

5. Serve warm.

Apple Pumpkin Butter

Prep time: 12 mins, Cook Time: 10 mins, Servings: 6

- 30 oz. pumpkin purée
- 4 apples, cored, peeled, and cubed
- 12 oz. apple cider

- 1 cup sugar
- 1 tbsp. pumpkin pie spice

1. In the Instant Pot, stir together the pumpkin purée with apples, apple cider, sugar, and pumpkin pie spice.
2. Lock the lid. Select the Manual mode and cook for 10 minutes at High Pressure.
3. Once cooking is complete, do a quick pressure release. Carefully open the lid.
4. Remove from the pot and serve in bowls.

Pumpkin Oatmeal

Prep time: 5 minutes | Cook time: 10 minutes | Serves 6
3 cups water
1½ cups 2% milk
1¼ cups steel-cut oats
3 tablespoons brown sugar
1½ teaspoons pumpkin pie spice
1 teaspoon ground cinnamon
¾ teaspoon salt
1 (15-ounce / 425-g) can solid-pack pumpkin

1. Place all the ingredients except the pumpkin into the Instant Pot and stir to incorporate.
2. Secure the lid. Select the Manual mode and set the cooking time for 10 minutes at High Pressure.
3. Once cooking is complete, do a natural pressure release for 10 minutes, then release any remaining pressure. Carefully open the lid.
4. Add the pumpkin and stir well. Allow the oatmeal to sit for 5 to 10 minutes to thicken. Serve immediately.

Carrot and Pineapple Oatmeal

Prep time: 10 minutes | Cook time: 10 minutes | Serves 8
4½ cups water
2 cups shredded carrots
1 cup steel-cut oats
1 (20-ounce/ 567-g) can crushed pineapple, undrained
1 cup raisins
1 teaspoon pumpkin pie spice
2 teaspoons ground cinnamon
Brown sugar (optional)
Cooking spray

1. Spray the bottom of the Instant Pot with cooking spray.
2. Combine the remaining ingredients except the brown sugar in the Instant Pot.
3. Secure the lid. Select the Manual mode and set the cooking time for 10 minutes at High Pressure.
4. Once cooking is complete, do a natural pressure release for 10 minutes, then release any remaining pressure. Carefully open the lid.
5. Serve sprinkled with the brown sugar, if desired.

Spiced Fruit Medley

Prep time: 5 minutes | Cook time: 1 minute | Serves 6
1 pound (454 g) frozen pineapple chunks
1 pound (454 g) sliced frozen peaches
1 cup frozen and pitted dark sweet cherries
2 ripe pears, sliced
¼ cup pure maple syrup
1 teaspoon curry powder, plus more as needed

1. Combine all the ingredients in the Instant Pot.
2. Secure the lid. Select the Manual mode and set the cooking time for 1 minute at High Pressure.
3. Once cooking is complete, do a quick pressure release. Carefully open the lid.
4. Stir the mixture well, adding more curry powder if you like it spicy. Serve warm.

Rhubarb Compote

Prep time: 10 minutes | Cook time: 3 minutes | Serves 6
Compote:
2 cups finely chopped fresh rhubarb
¼ cup sugar
⅓ cup water
For Serving:
3 cups reduced-fat plain Greek yogurt
2 tablespoons honey
¾ cup sliced almonds, toasted

1. Combine the rhubarb, sugar, and water in the Instant Pot.
2. Secure the lid. Select the Manual mode and set the cooking time for 3 minutes at High Pressure.

3. Once cooking is complete, do a natural pressure release for 10 minutes, then release any remaining pressure. Carefully open the lid.

4. Transfer the mixture to a bowl and let rest for a few minutes until cooled slightly. Place in the refrigerator until chilled.

5. When ready, whisk the yogurt and honey in a small bowl until well combined. Spoon into serving dishes and top each dish evenly with the compote. Scatter with the almonds and serve immediately.

Hard-Boiled Eggs

Prep time: 5 minutes | Cook time: 5 minutes | Serves 6
½ cup water
6 eggs

1. Place the trivet in the Instant Pot and pour in the water.

2. Crack each egg into a silicone cup. Carefully place the cups on top of the trivet.

3. Set the lid in place. Select the Manual mode and set the cooking time for 5 minutes on High Pressure. When the timer goes off, perform a quick pressure release. Carefully open the lid.

4. Carefully remove the cups from the pot. Use a spoon to pop the eggs out of the cups. Serve immediately.

Stone Fruit Compote

Prep time: 5 minutes | Cook time: 3 minutes | Makes about 2 cups
4 cups sliced stone fruit (plums, apricots, or peaches)
⅛ cup water
1 tablespoon pure maple syrup, plus additional as needed
1 tablespoon fresh lemon juice
½ teaspoon vanilla bean paste or extract
Pinch of ground cinnamon

1. Stir together all the ingredients in the Instant Pot.

2. Lock the lid. Select the Manual mode and set the cooking time for 1 minute at High Pressure.

3. When the timer beeps, perform a natural pressure release for 10 minutes, then release any remaining pressure. Carefully remove the lid.

4. Allow to simmer on Sauté for 2 minutes, stirring, or until thickened.

5. Taste and add additional maple syrup, as needed. Serve warm.

Special White Pancake

Prep time: 12 mins, Cook Time: 30 mins, Servings: 4
- 2½ tsps. baking powder
- 2 eggs, beaten
- 2 tbsps. sugar
- 1½ cups milk
- 2 cups white flour

1. In a bowl, mix the flour with eggs, milk, sugar, and baking powder. Stir to incorporate.

2. Spread out the mixture onto the bottom of the Instant Pot.

3. Lock the lid. Select the Manual mode and cook for 30 minutes at High Pressure.

4. Once cooking is complete, do a quick pressure release. Carefully open the lid.

5. Let the pancake cool for a few minutes before slicing to serve.

Bacon and Spinach Quiche

Prep time: 5 minutes | Cook time: 35 minutes | Serves 3
1 cup filtered water
5 eggs, lightly beaten
½ cup spinach, chopped
½ cup full-fat coconut milk
½ cup shredded full-fat Cheddar cheese
2 slices no-sugar-added bacon, cooked and finely chopped
½ teaspoon dried parsley
½ teaspoon dried basil
½ teaspoon freshly ground black pepper
¼ teaspoon kosher salt

1. Pour the water into the the Instant Pot, then place the trivet.

2. Stir together the remaining ingredients in a baking dish. Cover the dish loosely with aluminum foil. Place the dish on top of the trivet.

3. Secure the lid. Select the Manual mode and set the cooking time for 35 minutes at High Pressure.

4. Once cooking is complete, do a natural pressure release for 10 minutes, then release any remaining pressure. Carefully open the lid.

5. Serve warm.

Orange and Strawberry Compote

Prep time: 10 minutes, Cook Time: 15 minutes, Servings: 4

- 2 lbs. fresh strawberries, rinsed, trimmed, and cut in half
- 2 oz. fresh orange juice
- 1 vanilla bean, chopped
- ½ tsp. ground ginger
- ¼ cup sugar
- Toast, for serving

1. Put all the ingredients into the Instant Pot. Stir to mix well.

2. Lock the lid. Set to the Manual Mode, then set the timer for 15 minutes at High Pressure.

3. When the timer goes off, perform a natural pressure release for 10 minutes. Carefully open the lid.

4. Allow to cool and thicken before serving with the toast.

Strawberry and Pumpkin Spice Quinoa Bowl

Prep time: 12 minutes, Cook Time: 2 minutes, Servings: 4

- 2¼ cups water
- 2 tbsps. honey
- 2 cups chopped strawberries
- ¼ tsp. pumpkin pie spice
- 1 ½ cups quinoa

1. In the Instant Pot, mix the quinoa with honey, water, spice, and strawberries. Stir to combine.

2. Lock the lid. Select the Manual mode and set the cooking time for 2 minutes at High Pressure.

3. Once cooking is complete, do a natural pressure release for 10 minutes, then release any remaining pressure. Carefully open the lid.

4. Let the quinoa rest for 10 minutes. Give a good stir and serve immediately.

Coconut Muesli Stuffed Apples

Prep time: 10 minutes | Cook time: 3 minutes | Serves 2

⅓ cup water
2 large unpeeled organic apples, cored and tops removed
Filling:
½ cup coconut muesli
2 tablespoons butter, cubed
½ teaspoon ground cinnamon
2 teaspoons packed brown sugar

1. Pour the water into the Instant Pot and set aside.

2. Mix together all the ingredients for the filling in a bowl, mashing gently with a fork until incorporated.

3. Stuff each apple evenly with the muesli mixture, then arrange them in the Instant Pot.

4. Lock the lid. Select the Manual mode and set the cooking time for 3 minutes at Low Pressure, depending on how large the apples are.

5. Once cooking is complete, do a natural pressure release for 10 minutes, then release any remaining pressure. Carefully open the lid.

6. Let the apples cool for 5 minutes and serve.

Sweet Potato and Kale Egg Bites

Prep time: 7 minutes | Cook time: 20 minutes | Makes 7 egg bites

1 (14-ounce / 397-g) package firm tofu, lightly pressed
¼ cup coconut milk
¼ cup nutritional yeast
1 tablespoon cornstarch
½ to 1 teaspoon sea salt
½ teaspoon onion powder
½ teaspoon garlic powder
½ teaspoon ground turmeric
½ cup shredded sweet potato
Handful kale leaves, chopped small
1 cup plus 1 tablespoon water, divided
Freshly ground black pepper, to taste
Nonstick cooking spray

1. Lightly spray a silicone egg bites mold with nonstick cooking spray. Set aside.
2. Combine the tofu, milk, yeast, cornstarch, sea salt, onion powder, garlic powder, and turmeric in a food processor. Pulse until smooth.
3. Press the Sauté button to heat your Instant Pot until hot.
4. Add the sweet potato, kale, and 1 tablespoon of water. Sauté for 1 to 2 minutes. Stir the veggies into the tofu mixture and spoon the mixture into the prepared mold. Cover it tightly with aluminum foil and place on a trivet.
5. Pour the remaining 1 cup of water into the Instant Pot and insert the trivet.
6. Lock the lid. Select the Manual mode and set the cooking time for 18 minutes at High Pressure.
7. When the timer beeps, perform a natural pressure release for 10 minutes, then release any remaining pressure. Carefully remove the lid.
8. Remove the silicone mold from the Instant Pot and pull off the foil. Allow to cool for 5 minutes on the trivet. The bites will continue to firm as they cool.
9. Season to taste with pepper and serve warm.

Tex Mex Tofu Scramble

Prep time: 5 minutes | Cook time: 10 minutes | Serves 4
1 tablespoon olive oil
3 cloves garlic, minced
1 cup chopped red bell pepper
¼ cup canned green chilies, chopped
1 teaspoon ground cumin
1 teaspoon paprika
1 teaspoon chili powder
½ teaspoon salt
½ teaspoon black pepper
1 package extra firm tofu, cubed
1 cup fresh corn kernels
1 cup diced tomatoes
¼ cup vegetable broth or water
1 avocado, sliced
¼ cup chopped fresh cilantro (optional)
1. Set your Instant Pot to Sauté and heat the olive oil.

2. Add the garlic, red bell pepper, green chilies, cumin, paprika, chili powder, salt, and black pepper, stirring well, and sauté for 5 minutes.
3. Stir in the remaining ingredients, except for the avocado and cilantro.
4. Lock the lid. Select the Manual mode and set the cooking time for 4 minutes at High Pressure.
5. When the timer beeps, perform a quick pressure release. Carefully remove the lid and stir.
6. Serve garnished with avocado slices and fresh cilantro (if desired).

Tropical Fruit Chutney

Prep time: 5 minutes | Cook time: 20 minutes | Serves 6
2 mangoes, chopped
1 medium-sized pear, peeled and chopped
1 papaya, chopped
1 cup apple cider vinegar
½ cup brown sugar
¼ cup golden raisins
2 tablespoons fresh grated ginger
2 teaspoons lemon zest
½ teaspoon coriander
½ teaspoon cinnamon
¼ teaspoon cardamom
1. Stir together all the ingredients in the Instant Pot.
2. Secure the lid. Select the Manual mode and set the cooking time for 6 minutes at High Pressure.
3. Once cooking is complete, do a natural pressure release for 20 minutes, then release any remaining pressure. Carefully open the lid.
4. Press the Sauté button on the Instant Pot. Cook the chutney, stirring, for approximately 12 to 15 minutes, or until thickened. Serve warm.

Vanilla Applesauce

Prep time: 10 minutes | Cook time: 3 minutes | Makes 5 cups
7 medium apples (about 3 pounds / 1.4 kg), peeled and cored
½ cup water
½ cup sugar

1 tablespoon lemon juice

¼ teaspoon vanilla extract

1.   Slice each apple into 8 wedges on your cutting board, then slice each wedge crosswise in half.

2.   Add the apples to the Instant Pot along with the remaining ingredients. Stir well.

3.   Secure the lid. Select the Manual mode and set the cooking time for 3 minutes at High Pressure.

4.   Once cooking is complete, do a natural pressure release for 10 minutes, then release any remaining pressure. Carefully open the lid.

5.   Blend the mixture with an immersion blender until your desired consistency is achieved.

6.   Serve warm.

Veggie Quiche

Prep time: 12 mins, Cook Time: 20 mins, Servings: 6

- ½ cup milk
- 1 red bell pepper, chopped
- 2 green onions, chopped
- Salt, to taste
- 8 whisked eggs
- 1 cup water

1.   In a bowl, combine the whisked eggs with milk, bell pepper, onions and salt, and stir well. Pour the egg mixture into a pan.

2.   In your Instant Pot, add the water and trivet. Place the pan on the trivet and cover with tin foil.

3.   Lock the lid. Select the Manual mode and cook for 20 minutes at High Pressure.

4.   Once cooking is complete, do a quick pressure release. Carefully open the lid.

5.   Slice the quiche and divide between plates to serve.

Western Omelet

Prep time: 12 mins, Cook Time: 30 mins, Servings: 4

- ½ cup half-and-half
- 4 chopped spring onions
- 6 whisked eggs
- ¼ tsp. salt
- 8 oz. bacon, chopped
- 1½ cups water

1.   Place the steamer basket in the Instant Pot and pour in 1½ cups water.

2.   In a bowl, combine the eggs with half-and-half, bacon, spring onions and salt, and whisk well. Pour the egg mixture into a soufflé dish and transfer to the steamer basket.

3.   Lock the lid. Select the Steam mode and cook for 30 minutes at High Pressure.

4.   Once cooking is complete, do a quick pressure release. Carefully open the lid.

5.   Allow to cool for 5 minutes before serving.

CHAPTER 3 VEGETABLES

Broccoli Stuffed Potatoes

Prep time: 10 minutes | Cook time: 20 minutes | Serves 4

1 cup water

1 head broccoli, cut into florets

4 small russet potatoes

¾ cup half-and-half

1 tablespoon butter

2 cups Gruyere cheese, grated

1 teaspoon cornstarch

¼ cup chopped fresh chives

1. Pour the water in the Instant Pot and fit in a steamer basket.

2. Add the broccoli. Seal the lid. Select the Manual mode and set the cooking time for 1 minute at High Pressure.

3. Once cooking is complete, do a quick pressure release, then unlock the lid and transfer the broccoli to a bowl.

4. In the steamer basket, place the potatoes. Seal the lid again. Select the Manual mode and set the cooking time for 15 minutes on High Pressure.

5. Once cooking is complete, do a quick pressure release. Unlock the lid and let the potatoes cool.

6. Take out the steamer basket and discard the water. Press the Sauté button and warm half-and-half and butter until the butter melts.

7. In a bowl, mix the cheese with cornstarch and pour the mixture into the pot. Stir until the cheese melts. Transfer the mixture in a large bowl.

8. Toss the broccoli with the mixture to combine well. Cut a slit into each potato and stuff with the broccoli mixture. Scatter with chives to serve.

Baked Cabbage with Pepper

Prep time: 15 minutes | Cook time: 25 minutes | Serves 2

1 tablespoon olive oil, divided

½ pound (227 g) green cabbage, shredded

1 garlic clove, sliced

1 onion, thinly sliced

1 Serrano pepper, chopped

1 sweet pepper, thinly sliced

Sea salt and ground black pepper, to taste

1 teaspoon paprika

1 cup cream of mushroom soup

4 ounces (113 g) Colby cheese, shredded

1 cup water

1. Grease a baking dish with ½ tablespoon of olive oil. Add the cabbage, garlic, onion, and peppers. Stir to combine.

2. Drizzle with remaining oil and season with salt, black pepper, and paprika. Pour in the mushroom soup. Top with the shredded cheese and cover with aluminum foil.

3. Pour the water in the Instant Pot and fit in a trivet. Lower the dish onto the trivet.

4. Secure the lid. Choose the Manual mode and set the cooking time for 25 minutes at High pressure.

5. Once cooking is complete, perform a quick pressure release. Carefully open the lid. Serve warm.

Spaghetti Squash with Spinach

Prep time: 10 minutes | Cook time: 8 minutes | Serves 4

1 large spaghetti squash, cut into 8 pieces

1½ cups water

3 tablespoons olive oil

8 cloves garlic, thinly sliced

½ cup slivered almonds

1 teaspoon red pepper flakes

4 cups chopped fresh spinach

1 teaspoon kosher salt

1 cup shredded Parmesan cheese

1. Pour the water into the Instant Pot. Put a trivet in the pot. Set the squash on the trivet.

2. Lock the lid. Select Manual mode and set the timer for 7 minutes on High Pressure.

3. When timer beeps, perform a natural pressure release for 10 minutes, then release any remaining pressure.

4. Remove the squash, and cut it in half lengthwise. Use a fork to scrape the strands of one half into a large bowl. Measure out 4 cups. Reserve the other half for other use.

5. Set the squash shell aside to use as a serving vessel. Clean the pot.

6. Select Sauté mode. When the pot is hot, add the olive oil. Once the oil is hot, add the garlic, almonds, and pepper flakes. Cook, stirring constantly and being careful not to burn the garlic for 1 minute.

7. Add the spinach, salt, and spaghetti squash. Stir well to thoroughly combine ingredients until the spinach wilts.

8. Transfer the mixture to the reserved squash shell. Sprinkle with the Parmesan cheese before serving.

Pecan and Cherry Stuffed Pumpkin

Prep time: 20 minutes | Cook time: 20 minutes | Serves 4

1 (2-pound / 907-g) pumpkin, halved lengthwise, stems trimmed
2 tablespoons olive oil
1 cup water
½ cup dried cherries
1 teaspoon dried parsley
5 toasted bread slices, cubed
1 teaspoon onion powder
1½ cups vegetable broth
Salt and black pepper, to taste
½ cup chopped pecans, for topping

1. Brush the pumpkin with olive oil. Pour the water in the Instant Pot and fit in a trivet. Place the pumpkin, skin-side down, on the trivet.

2. Seal the lid. Select the Manual mode and set the cooking time for 15 minutes at High Pressure.

3. Once cooking is complete, do a quick pressure release. Carefully open the lid.

4. Remove the pumpkin and water. Press the Sauté button, add the remaining ingredients. Stir for 5 minutes or until the liquid is reduced by half.

5. Divide the mixture between pumpkin halves and top with pecans.

Cauliflower and Tomato Curry

Prep time: 10 minutes | Cook time: 2 minutes | Serves 4 to 6

1 medium head cauliflower, cut into bite-size pieces
1 (14-ounce / 397-g) can sugar-free diced tomatoes, undrained
1 bell pepper, thinly sliced
1 (14-ounce / 397-g) can full-fat coconut milk
½ to 1 cup water
2 tablespoons red curry paste
1 teaspoon salt
1 teaspoon garlic powder
½ teaspoon onion powder
½ teaspoon ground ginger
¼ teaspoon chili powder
Freshly ground black pepper, to taste

1. Add all the ingredients, except for the black pepper, to the Instant Pot and stir to combine.

2. Lock the lid. Select the Manual setting and set the cooking time for 2 minutes at High Pressure. Once the timer goes off, use a quick pressure release. Carefully open the lid.

3. Sprinkle the black pepper and stir well. Serve immediately.

Green Beans with Toasted Peanuts

Prep time: 10 minutes | Cook time: 1 minutes | Serves 4

1 cup water
1 pound (454 g) green beans, trimmed
1 lemon, juiced
2 tablespoons olive oil
Salt and black pepper, to taste
2 tablespoons toasted peanuts

1. Pour the water in the Instant Pot, then fit in a steamer basket and arrange the green beans on top.

2. Seal the lid. Select the Manual mode and set the time for 1 minute on High Pressure.

3. Once cooking is complete, do a quick pressure release. Unlock the lid.

4. Transfer the green beans onto a plate and mix in lemon juice, olive oil, salt, pepper, and toasted peanuts. Serve immediately.

Khoreshe Karafs

Prep time: 20 minutes | Cook time: 11 minutes | Serves 2

1 tablespoon unsalted butter
½ onion, chopped
1 garlic clove, minced
½ pound (227 g) celery stalks, diced
1 Persian lime, prick a few holes
1 tablespoon fresh cilantro, roughly chopped
1 tablespoon fresh mint, finely chopped
½ teaspoon mustard seeds
2 cups vegetable broth
½ teaspoon cayenne pepper
Sea salt and ground black pepper, to taste

1. Press the Sauté button of the Instant Pot. Add and melt the butter.
2. Add and sauté the onions and garlic for about 3 minutes or until tender and fragrant.
3. Stir in the remaining ingredients, except for the basmati rice.
4. Secure the lid. Choose the Manual mode and set the cooking time for 18 minutes at High pressure.
5. Once cooking is complete, use a natural pressure release for 15 minutes, then release any remaining pressure. Carefully open the lid.
6. Serve hot.

Honey Carrot Salad

Prep time: 10 minutes | Cook time: 3 minutes | Serves 2 to 4

1 cup water
1 pound (454 g) carrots, sliced to 2-inch chunks
1 scallion, finely sliced
½ tablespoon Dijon mustard
½ tablespoon lime juice
1 teaspoon honey
¼ teaspoon red pepper flakes
½ teaspoon Himalayan salt
¼ teaspoon ground white pepper
1 tablespoon olive oil

1. Pour the water in the Instant Pot and fit in a steamer basket. Place the carrots in the steamer basket.
2. Secure the lid. Choose the Steam mode and set the cooking time for 3 minutes at High pressure.
3. Once cooking is complete, perform a quick pressure release. Carefully open the lid.
4. Toss the carrots with the remaining ingredients in a serving bowl and serve chilled.

Artichokes with Onion

Prep time: 6 mins, Cook time: 30 mins, Servings: 8

- ½ cup organic chicken broth
- Salt and pepper, to taste
- 4 large artichokes, trimmed and cleaned
- 1 onion, chopped
- 1 garlic clove, crushed

1. Place all ingredients in the Instant Pot.
2. Lock the lid. Set the Instant Pot to Manual mode, then set the timer for 30 minutes at High Pressure.
3. Once cooking is complete, do a quick pressure release. Carefully open the lid.
4. Serve the artichokes with lemon juice.

Garlicky Baby Bok Choy

Prep time: 9 mins, Cook time: 4 mins, Servings: 6

- 1 tsp. peanut oil
- 1 lb. baby Bok choy, trimmed and washed
- Salt and pepper, to taste
- 4 garlic cloves, minced
- 1 tsp. red pepper flakes
- 1 cup water

1. Press the Sauté button on the Instant Pot.
2. Heat the oil and sauté the garlic for 1 minute until fragrant.
3. Add the Bok choy and sprinkle salt and pepper for seasoning.
4. Pour in the water.
5. Lock the lid. Set the Instant Pot to Manual mode, then set the timer for 4 minutes at High Pressure.
6. Once cooking is complete, do a quick pressure release. Carefully open the lid.
7. Sprinkle with red pepper flakes, then serve.

Mushrooms with Garlic

Prep time: 12 mins, Cook Time: 10 mins, Servings: 1

- ½ cup water
- 4 oz. mushrooms, sliced
- 2 garlic cloves, minced
- 1 tbsp. olive oil
- Salt and pepper, to taste

1. Pour water along with mushrooms in an Instant Pot.
2. Lock the lid. Set the Instant Pot to Manual mode, then set the timer for 5 minutes at High Pressure.
3. Once cooking is complete, do a quick pressure release. Carefully open the lid.
4. Drain the mushroom and then return back to the Instant Pot.
5. Now add olive oil to the pot and mix.
6. Press the Sauté function of the pot and let it cook for 3 minutes.
7. Sauté every 30 seconds.
8. Add the garlic and sauté for 2 minutes or until fragrant. Sprinkle with salt and pepper, then serve the dish.

Steamed Asparagus

Prep time: 5mins, Cook time: 5 mins, Servings: 1

- 7 asparagus spears, washed and trimmed
- ¼ tsp. pepper
- 1 tbsp. extra virgin olive oil
- Juice from freshly squeezed ¼ lemon
- ¼ tsp. salt
- 1 cup water

1. Place a trivet or the steamer rack in the Instant Pot and pour in the water.
2. In a mixing bowl, combine the asparagus spears, salt, pepper, and lemon juice.
3. Place on top of the trivet.
4. Lock the lid. Set the Instant Pot to Steam mode, then set the timer for 5 minutes at High Pressure.
5. Once cooking is complete, do a quick pressure release. Carefully open the lid.
6. Drizzle the asparagus with olive oil.

Veggie Stew

Prep time: 6 mins, Cook time: 10 mins, Servings: 5

- ½ cup chopped tomatoes
- 1 stalk celery, minced
- 2 zucchinis, chopped
- 1 lb. mushrooms, sliced
- 1 onion, chopped
- Salt and pepper, to taste

1. Place all ingredients in the Instant Pot.
2. Pour in enough water until half of the vegetables are submerged.
3. Lock the lid. Set the Instant Pot to Manual mode, then set the timer for 10 minutes at High Pressure.
4. Once cooking is complete, do a quick pressure release. Carefully open the lid.
5. Serve warm.

Zucchini Sticks

Prep time: 5 minutes | Cook time: 8 minutes | Serves 2

2 zucchinis, trimmed and cut into sticks
2 teaspoons olive oil
½ teaspoon white pepper
½ teaspoon salt
1 cup water

1. Place the zucchini sticks in the Instant Pot pan and sprinkle with the olive oil, white pepper and salt.
2. Pour the water and put the trivet in the pot. Place the pan on the trivet.
3. Lock the lid. Select the Manual setting and set the cooking time for 8 minutes at High Pressure. Once the timer goes off, use a quick pressure release. Carefully open the lid.
4. Remove the zucchinis from the pot and serve.

Ratatouille

Prep time: 20 mins, Cook Time: 10 mins, Servings: 4

- 2 cups water
- 2 medium zucchini, sliced
- 3 tomatoes, sliced
- 2 eggplants, sliced
- 1 tbsp. olive oil
- Salt and pepper, to taste

1. Pour the water into the Instant Pot.
2. In a baking dish, arrange a layer of the zucchini.
3. Top with a layer of the tomatoes.
4. Place a layer of eggplant slices on top.
5. Continue layering until you use all the ingredients.
6. Drizzle with olive oil.
7. Place the baking dish on the trivet and lower it.
8. Lock the lid. Set the Instant Pot to Manual mode, then set the timer for 10 minutes at High Pressure.
9. Once cooking is complete, do a quick pressure release. Carefully open the lid.
10. Sprinkle with salt and pepper and serve warm!

Italian Carrot and Potato Medley

Prep time: 15 minutes | Cook time: 11 minutes | Serves 4

2 tablespoons olive oil
1 cup potatoes, peeled and chopped
3 carrots, peeled and chopped
3 garlic cloves, minced
1 cup vegetable broth
1 teaspoon Italian seasoning
Salt and black pepper, to taste
1 tablespoon chopped parsley
1 tablespoon chopped oregano

1. Set the Instant Pot to the Sauté mode. Heat the olive oil until shimmering.
2. Add and sauté the potatoes and carrots for 5 minutes or until tender.
3. Add the garlic and cook for a minute or until fragrant. Pour in the vegetable broth, season with Italian seasoning, salt, and black pepper.
4. Seal the lid. Select the Manual mode and set the time for 5 minutes at High Pressure.
5. Once cooking is complete, do a quick pressure release, then unlock the lid.
6. Spoon the potatoes and carrots into a serving bowl and mix in the parsley and oregano. Serve warm.

Lush Veg Medley

Prep time: 50 mins, Cook Time: 8 mins, Servings: 4

- 1 cup water

- 1 tbsp. raisins
- 1 zucchini, sliced
- 1 eggplant, cubed
- 3 tbsps. olive oil
- 10 halved cherry tomatoes
- 2 potatoes, cubed
- 2 tbsps. raisins

1. In the Instant Pot, add the water. Add the potatoes and zucchini.
2. Lock the lid. Set the Instant Pot to Manual mode, then set the timer for 8 minutes on High Pressure.
3. Once cooking is complete, do a quick pressure release. Carefully open the lid.
4. Drain water and add olive oil.
5. Mix in the tomatoes and eggplant. Let cook for 2 minutes.
6. Top with the raisins before serving.

Tomatillo and Jackfruit Tinga

Prep time: 15 minutes | Cook time: 21 minutes | Serves 4

1 tablespoon olive oil
1½ cups minced onion
6 cloves garlic, minced
2 tablespoons minced jalapeño
1 (20-ounce / 565-g) can jackfruit in brine, rinsed, shredded
1 (14.5-ounce / 411-g) can diced tomatoes
1 cup diced tomatillos
1½ teaspoons dried thyme
1 teaspoon dried oregano
¼ cup water
½ teaspoon ground cumin
Salt, to taste

1. Select the Sauté setting of the Instant Pot and heat the oil until shimmering.
2. Add the onion and sauté for 5 minutes or until transparent. Then add the garlic and jalapeño and sauté for 1 minute more.
3. Add the jackfruit, tomatoes, tomatillos, thyme, oregano, water, and cumin to the pot and stir to combine.
4. Put the lid on. Select the Manual setting and set the timer for 15 minutes on High Pressure.

5. When timer beeps, allow the pressure to release naturally for 5 minutes, then release any remaining pressure. Open the lid.

6. Sprinkle with salt and serve.

Ritzy Green Pea and Cauliflower Curry

Prep time: 20 minutes | Cook time: 8 minutes | Serves 4

3 large tomatoes

4 large cloves garlic

1-inch piece ginger

1 green chili

12 raw cashews

1½ tablespoons olive oil

1 bay leaf

3 green cardamoms

6 peppercorns

3 cloves

1 large red onion, chopped

1½ teaspoons coriander powder

1 teaspoon garam masala

½ teaspoon red chili powder

½ teaspoon turmeric powder

1 teaspoon salt

¼ cup plain yogurt, at room temperature

½ cup plus 2 tablespoons coconut milk

¼ cup water

1 large head cauliflower, cut into florets

½ cup frozen green peas Cilantro, for garnish

1. Using a blender, purée the tomatoes, garlic, ginger, green chili and cashews to a smooth paste. Set aside.

2. Press the Sauté button on the Instant Pot. Add the oil and then add the bay leaf, green cardamoms, peppercorns and cloves. Sauté for a few seconds until the spices are fragrant and then add the onion. Cook the onion until soft, around 2 minutes.

3. Add the puréed tomato mixture. Cook for 2 minutes and then add the coriander powder, garam masala, red chili powder, turmeric powder and salt. Stir to combine the spices and cook them for 30 seconds.

4. Add the yogurt, whisking continuously until well combined.

5. Add the coconut milk and the water and mix to combine.

6. Add the cauliflower florets and peas and toss to combine them with the masala.

7. Close the lid and press the Manual button. Set the timer for 3 minutes on Low Pressure.

8. When timer beeps, do a quick pressure release.

9. Open the pot, give them a stir. Garnish with cilantro and serve.

Satarash with Eggs

Prep time: 10 minutes | Cook time: 5 minutes | Serves 4

2 tablespoons olive oil

1 white onion, chopped

2 cloves garlic

2 ripe tomatoes, puréed

1 green bell pepper, deseeded and sliced

1 red bell pepper, deseeded and sliced

1 teaspoon paprika

½ teaspoon dried oregano

½ teaspoon turmeric

Kosher salt and ground black pepper, to taste

1 cup water

4 large eggs, lightly whisked

1. Press the Sauté button on the Instant Pot and heat the olive oil. Add the onion and garlic to the pot and sauté for 2 minutes, or until fragrant. Stir in the remaining ingredients, except for the eggs.

2. Lock the lid. Select the Manual mode and set the cooking time for 3 minutes on High Pressure. When the timer goes off, perform a quick pressure release. Carefully open the lid.

3. Fold in the eggs and stir to combine. Lock the lid and let it sit in the residual heat for 5 minutes. Serve warm.

Sautéed Brussels Sprouts And Pecans

Prep time: 4 mins, Cook time: 6 mins, Servings: 4

- ¼ cup chopped pecans
- 2 garlic cloves, minced
- Salt and pepper, to taste
- 2 tbsps. water
- 2 cups baby Brussels sprouts
- 1 tbsp. coconut oil

1. Press the Sauté button on the Instant Pot and heat the oil.
2. Sauté the garlic for 1 minute or until fragrant.
3. Add the Brussels sprouts. Sprinkle salt and pepper for seasoning.
4. Add the water.
5. Lock the lid. Set the Instant Pot to Manual mode, then set the timer for 3 minutes at High Pressure.
6. Once cooking is complete, do a quick pressure release. Carefully open the lid.
7. Add the pecans and set to the Sauté mode and sauté for 3 minutes or until the pecans are roasted.
8. Serve immediately.

Sesame Bok Choy

Prep time: 6 mins, Cook Time: 4 mins, Servings: 4
- 1 tsp. soy sauce
- ½ tsp. sesame oil
- 1½ cups water
- 1 medium Bok choy
- 2 tsps. sesame seeds
1. Pour the water into the Instant Pot.
2. Place the Bok choy inside the steamer basket.
3. Lower the basket
4. Lock the lid. Set the Instant Pot to Manual mode, then set the timer for 4 minutes at High Pressure.
5. Once cooking is complete, do a quick pressure release. Carefully open the lid.
6. In a serving bowl, set in the Bok choy. Toss with the remaining ingredients to coat.
7. Serve immediately!

Spaghetti Squash Noodles

Prep time: 5 minutes | Cook time: 18 minutes | Serves 4
2 pounds (907 g) spaghetti squash
1 cup water
3 garlic cloves
1 cup fresh basil leaves
½ cup olive oil
⅓ cup unsalted toasted almonds
¼ cup flat-leaf parsley
3 tablespoons grated Parmesan cheese

½ teaspoon fine grind sea salt
½ teaspoon ground black pepper
1. Using a knife, pierce all sides of the squash to allow the steam to penetrate during cooking.
2. Pour the water into the Instant Pot and put the trivet in the pot. Place the squash on the trivet.
3. Lock the lid. Select the Manual mode and set the cooking time for 18 minutes at High Pressure. When the timer goes off, use a natural pressure release for 10 minutes, then release any remaining pressure. Carefully open the lid.
4. Remove the trivet and squash from the pot. Set aside to cool for 15 minutes, or until the squash is cool enough to handle.
5. Make the pesto sauce by placing the remaining ingredients in a food processor. Pulse until the ingredients are well combined and form a thick paste. Set aside.
6. Cut the cooled spaghetti squash in half lengthwise. Using a spoon, scoop out and discard the seeds.
7. Using a fork, scrape the flesh of the squash to create the noodles. Transfer the noodles to a large bowl.
8. Divide the squash noodles among 4 serving bowls. Top each serving with the pesto sauce. Serve hot.

Spaghetti Squash Noodles with Tomatoes

Prep time: 15 minutes | Cook time: 14 to 16 minutes | Serves 4
1 medium spaghetti squash
1 cup water
2 tablespoons olive oil
1 small yellow onion, diced
6 garlic cloves, minced
2 teaspoons crushed red pepper flakes
2 teaspoons dried oregano
1 cup sliced cherry tomatoes
1 teaspoon kosher salt
½ teaspoon freshly ground black pepper
1 (14.5-ounce / 411-g) can sugar-free crushed tomatoes
¼ cup capers
1 tablespoon caper brine

½ cup sliced olives

1. With a sharp knife, halve the spaghetti squash crosswise. Using a spoon, scoop out the seeds and sticky gunk in the middle of each half.
2. Pour the water into the Instant Pot and place the trivet in the pot with the handles facing up. Arrange the squash halves, cut side facing up, on the trivet.
3. Lock the lid. Select the Manual mode and set the cooking time for 7 minutes on High Pressure. When the timer goes off, use a quick pressure release. Carefully open the lid.
4. Remove the trivet and pour out the water that has collected in the squash cavities. Using the tines of a fork, separate the cooked strands into spaghetti-like pieces and set aside in a bowl.
5. Pour the water out of the pot. Select the Sauté mode and heat the oil.
6. Add the onion to the pot and sauté for 3 minutes. Add the garlic, pepper flakes and oregano to the pot and sauté for 1 minute.
7. Stir in the cherry tomatoes, salt and black pepper and cook for 2 minutes, or until the tomatoes are tender.
8. Pour in the crushed tomatoes, capers, caper brine and olives and bring the mixture to a boil. Continue to cook for 2 to 3 minutes to allow the flavors to meld.
9. Stir in the spaghetti squash noodles and cook for 1 to 2 minutes to warm everything through.
10. Transfer the dish to a serving platter and serve.

Spinach with Almonds and Olives

Prep time: 15 minutes | Cook time: 2 to 3 minutes | Serves 4
1 tablespoon olive oil
3 cloves garlic, smashed
Bunch scallions, chopped
2 pounds (907 g) spinach, washed
1 cup vegetable broth
1 tablespoon champagne vinegar
½ teaspoon dried dill weed
¼ teaspoon cayenne pepper
Seasoned salt and ground black pepper, to taste
½ cup almonds, soaked overnight and drained
2 tablespoons green olives, pitted and halved

2 tablespoons water
1 tablespoon extra-virgin olive oil
2 teaspoons lemon juice
1 teaspoon garlic powder
1 teaspoon onion powder

1. Press the Sauté button on the Instant Pot and heat the olive oil. Add the garlic and scallions to the pot and sauté for 1 to 2 minutes, or until fragrant.
2. Stir in the spinach, vegetable broth, vinegar, dill, cayenne pepper, salt and black pepper.
3. Lock the lid. Select the Manual mode and set the cooking time for 1 minute on High Pressure. When the timer goes off, perform a quick pressure release. Carefully open the lid.
4. Stir in the remaining ingredients.
5. Transfer to serving plates and serve immediately.

Tofu and Mango Curry

Prep time: 15 minutes | Cook time: 9 minutes | Serves 2
8 ounces (227 g) extra-firm tofu, pressed to remove the moisture, cubed
¼ teaspoon smoked paprika
¼ teaspoon crushed red pepper
1¼ teaspoon salt, divided
⅛ teaspoon ground black pepper
2 tablespoons olive oil, divided
½ teaspoon mustard seeds
2 dried red chilies
½ medium white onion, diced
1½-inch piece ginger, grated
¾ cup gresh mango purée
½ cup coconut milk
1 teaspoon curry powder
½ cup water
Juice of ½ lemon
Cilantro, to garnish

1. Toss the tofu cubes with smoked paprika, crushed red pepper, ¼ teaspoon salt and ground black pepper.
2. Press the Sauté button on the Instant Pot. Add 1 tablespoon of oil to the pot, then add the spiced tofu cubes and cook for 4 minutes, or until lightly browned on all sides. Remove the tofu cubes to a bowl and set aside.

3. Add another tablespoon of oil to the pot, then add the mustard seeds. Let the mustard seeds pop and then add the dried red chilies. Sauté for a few seconds, then add the onion and ginger. Cook the onion and ginger for a minute until the onion turns a little soft.

4. Add the mango purée, coconut milk, and curry powder, then add 1 teaspoon of salt and let it all cook for a minute.

5. Add the water along with the sautéed tofu cubes and close the lid. Press the Manual button and set the timer for 3 minutes on High Pressure.

6. When timer beeps, do a quick pressure release. Open the lid.

7. Stir in the lemon juice, then transfer the curry to a serving bowl. Garnish with cilantro and serve.

Vegetarian Mac and Cheese

Prep time: 30 mins, Cook time: 4 mins, Servings: 10

- 4 cups water
- 1 tsp. garlic powder
- 16 oz. elbow macaroni pasta
- Salt and pepper, to taste
- 2 cups frozen mixed vegetables
- 1 cup shredded Cheddar
- 1 cup milk
- Fresh parsley, for garnish

1. To the Instant Pot, add the water, garlic powder and pasta. Sprinkle with salt and pepper.

2. Lock the lid. Set the Instant Pot to Manual mode, then set the timer for 4 minutes at High Pressure.

3. Once cooking is complete, do a quick pressure release. Carefully open the lid.

4. Add the vegetables, Cheddar and milk, then cover the pot and press Sauté.

5. Simmer until the vegetables have softened.

6. Garnish with fresh parsley and serve.

Vegetarian Smothered Cajun Greens

Prep time: 6 mins, Cook time: 3 mins, Servings: 4

- 2 tsps. crushed garlic
- Salt and pepper, to taste
- 1 onion, chopped

- 6 cups raw greens
- 1 tbsp. coconut oil
- 1 cup water

1. Press the Sauté button on the Instant Pot and heat the coconut oil.

2. Sauté the onion and garlic for 2 minutes or until fragrant.

3. Add the greens and Sprinkle salt and pepper for seasoning.

4. Add the water.

5. Lock the lid. Set the Instant Pot to Manual mode, then set the timer for 3 minutes at High Pressure.

6. Once cooking is complete, do a quick pressure release. Carefully open the lid.

7. Sprinkle with red chili flakes, then serve.

Vinegary Broccoli with Cheese

Prep time: 5 minutes | Cook time: 5 minutes | Serves 4

1 pound (454 g) broccoli, cut into florets
1 cup water
2 garlic cloves, minced
1 cup crumbled Cottage cheese
2 tablespoons balsamic vinegar
1 teaspoon cumin seeds
1 teaspoon mustard seeds
Salt and pepper, to taste

1. Pour the water into the Instant Pot and put the steamer basket in the pot. Place the broccoli in the steamer basket.

2. Close and secure the lid. Select the Manual setting and set the cooking time for 5 minutes at High Pressure. Once the timer goes off, do a quick pressure release. Carefully open the lid.

3. Stir in the remaining ingredients.

4. Serve immediately.

Zoodles with Mediterranean Sauce

Prep time: 10 minutes | Cook time: 5 minutes | Serves 2

1 tablespoon olive oil
2 tomatoes, chopped
½ cup water
½ cup roughly chopped fresh parsley

3 tablespoons ground almonds
1 tablespoon fresh rosemary, chopped
1 tablespoon apple cider vinegar
1 teaspoon garlic, smashed
2 zucchinis, spiralized and cooked
½ avocado, pitted and sliced
Salt and ground black pepper, to taste

1. Add the olive oil, tomatoes, water, parsley, ground almonds, rosemary, apple cider vinegar and garlic to the Instant Pot.
2. Lock the lid. Select the Manual mode and set the cooking time for 5 minutes on High Pressure. When the timer beeps, perform a natural pressure release for 10 minutes, then release any remaining pressure. Carefully open the lid.
3. Divide the cooked zucchini spirals between two serving plates. Spoon the sauce over each serving. Top with the avocado slices and season with salt and black pepper.
4. Serve immediately.

Zucchini and Bell Pepper Stir Fry

Prep time: 6 mins, Cook time: 5 mins, Servings: 6

- 2 large zucchinis, sliced
- 1 tbsp. coconut oil
- 4 garlic cloves, minced
- 2 red sweet bell peppers, julienned
- 1 onion, chopped
- Salt and pepper, to taste
- ¼ cup water

1. Press the Sauté button on the Instant Pot.
2. Heat the coconut oil and sauté the onion and garlic for 2 minutes or until fragrant.
3. Add the zucchini and red bell peppers.
4. Sprinkle salt and pepper for seasoning.
5. Pour in the water.
6. Lock the lid. Set the Instant Pot to Manual mode, then set the timer for 5 minutes at High Pressure.
7. Once cooking is complete, do a quick pressure release. Carefully open the lid.
8. Serve warm.

Daikon and Zucchini Fritters

Prep time: 10 minutes | Cook time: 8 minutes | Serves 4
2 large zucchinis, grated
1 daikon, diced
1 egg, beaten
1 teaspoon ground flax meal
1 teaspoon salt
1 tablespoon coconut oil

1. In the mixing bowl, combine all the ingredients, except for the coconut oil. Form the zucchini mixture into fritters.
2. Press the Sauté button on the Instant Pot and melt the coconut oil.
3. Place the zucchini fritters in the hot oil and cook for 4 minutes on each side, or until golden brown.
4. Transfer to a plate and serve.

Zucchini and Tomato Melange

Prep time: 13 mins, Cook time: 10 mins, Servings: 4

- 5 garlic cloves, minced
- 3 medium zucchinis, chopped
- 1 lb. puréed tomatoes
- 1 onion, chopped
- 1 tbsp. coconut oil
- Salt and pepper, to taste
- 1 cup water

1. Place the tomatoes in a food processor and blend until smooth.
2. Press the Sauté button on the Instant Pot and heat the oil.
3. Sauté the garlic and onions for 2 minutes or until fragrant.
4. Add the zucchini and tomato purée.
5. Sprinkle salt and pepper for seasoning.
6. Add the water to add more moisture.
7. Lock the lid. Set the Instant Pot to Manual mode, then set the timer for 10 minutes at High Pressure.
8. Once cooking is complete, do a quick pressure release. Carefully open the lid.
9. Serve warm.

CHAPTER 4 FISH AND SEAFOOD

Tuna with Eggs

Prep time: 5 minutes | Cook time: 15 minutes | Serves 4

2 cans tuna, drained
2 eggs, beaten
1 can cream of celery soup
2 carrots, peeled and chopped
1 cup frozen peas
½ cup water
¾ cup milk
¼ cup diced onions
2 tablespoons butter
Salt and ground black pepper, to taste

1. Combine all the ingredients in the Instant Pot and stir to mix well.
2. Secure the lid. Select the Manual mode and set the cooking time for 15 minutes at High Pressure.
3. Once cooking is complete, do a quick pressure release. Carefully open the lid.
4. Divide the mix into bowls and serve.

Crispy Salmon Fillets

Prep time: 5 minutes | Cook time: 5 minutes | Serves 2

1 tablespoon avocado oil
2 (3-ounce / 85-g) salmon fillets
1 teaspoon paprika
½ teaspoon salt
¼ teaspoon dried thyme
¼ teaspoon onion powder
¼ teaspoon pepper
⅛ teaspoon cayenne pepper

1. Drizzle the avocado oil over salmon fillets. Combine the remaining ingredients in a small bowl and rub all over fillets.
2. Press the Sauté button on the Instant Pot. Add the salmon fillets and sear for 2 to 5 minutes until the salmon easily flakes with a fork.
3. Serve warm.

Salmon with Dijon Mustard

Prep time: 5 minutes | Cook time: 5 minutes | Serves 2

1 cup water
2 fish fillets or steaks, such as salmon, cod, or halibut (1-inch thick)
Salt and ground black pepper, to taste
2 teaspoons Dijon mustard

1. Add the water to the Instant Pot and insert a trivet.
2. Season the fish with salt and pepper to taste. Put the fillets, skin-side down, on the trivet and top with the Dijon mustard.
3. Secure the lid. Select the Manual mode and set the cooking time for 5 minutes at High Pressure.
4. Once cooking is complete, do a quick pressure release. Carefully open the lid.
5. Divide the fish between two plates and serve.

Salmon Packets

Prep time: 8 minutes | Cook time: 6 minutes | Serves 4

1½ cups cold water
4 (5-ounce / 142-g) salmon fillets
½ teaspoon fine sea salt
¼ teaspoon ground black pepper
1 lime, thinly sliced
4 teaspoons extra-virgin olive oil, divided
Fresh thyme leaves

1. Pour the cold water into the Instant Pot and insert a steamer basket.
2. Sprinkle the fish on all sides with the salt and pepper.
3. Take four sheets of parchment paper and place 3 lime slices on each sheet. Top the lime slices with a piece of fish.
4. Drizzle with 1 teaspoon of olive oil and place a few thyme leaves on top. Cover each fillet with the parchment by folding in the edges and folding down the top like an envelope to close tightly.
5. Stack the packets in the steamer basket, seam-side down.
6. Secure the lid. Select the Manual mode and set the cooking time for 6 minutes at Low Pressure.

7. When the timer beeps, perform a natural pressure release for 10 minutes, then release any remaining pressure. Carefully remove the lid.

8. Remove the fish packets from the pot.

9. Serve the fish garnished with the fresh thyme.

Steamed Salmon

Prep time: 5 minutes | Cook time: 10 minutes | Serves 2

1 cup water

2 salmon fillets

Salt and ground black pepper, to taste

1. Pour the water into the Instant Pot and add a trivet.

2. Season the salmon fillets with salt and black pepper to taste. Put the salmon fillets on the trivet.

3. Secure the lid. Select the Steam mode and set the cooking time for 10 minutes at High Pressure.

4. Once cooking is complete, do a natural pressure release for 10 minutes, then release any remaining pressure. Carefully open the lid.

5. Serve hot.

Salmon with Broccoli

Prep time: 5 minutes | Cook time: 5 minutes | Serves 2

1 cup water

8 ounces (227 g) salmon fillets

8 ounces (227 g) broccoli, cut into florets

Salt and ground black pepper, to taste

1. Pour the water into the Instant Pot and insert a trivet.

2. Season the salmon and broccoli florets with salt and pepper. Put them on the trivet.

3. Secure the lid. Select the Steam mode and set the cooking time for 5 minutes at High Pressure.

4. Once cooking is complete, do a natural pressure release for 10 minutes, then release any remaining pressure. Carefully open the lid.

5. Serve hot.

Pesto Fish Packets with Parmesan

Prep time: 8 minutes | Cook time: 6 minutes | Serves 4

1½ cups cold water.

4 (4-ounce / 113-g) white fish fillets, such as cod or haddock

1 teaspoon fine sea salt

½ teaspoon ground black pepper

1 (4-ounce / 113-g) jar pesto

½ cup shredded Parmesan cheese (about 2 ounces / 57 g)

Halved cherry tomatoes, for garnish

1. Pour the water into your Instant Pot and insert a steamer basket.

2. Sprinkle the fish on all sides with the salt and pepper. Take four sheets of parchment paper and place a fillet in the center of each sheet.

3. Dollop 2 tablespoons of the pesto on top of each fillet and sprinkle with 2 tablespoons of the Parmesan cheese.

4. Wrap the fish in the parchment by folding in the edges and folding down the top like an envelope to close tightly.

5. Stack the packets in the steamer basket, seam-side down.

6. Lock the lid. Select the Manual mode and set the cooking time for 6 minutes at Low Pressure.

7. Once cooking is complete, do a natural pressure release for 10 minutes, then release any remaining pressure. Carefully open the lid.

8. Remove the fish packets from the pot. Transfer to a serving plate and garnish with the cherry tomatoes.

9. Serve immediately.

Flounder Fillets with Capers

Prep time: 3 mins, Cook time: 10 mins, Servings: 4

- 1 cup water
- 1 tbsp. chopped fresh dill
- 4 lemon wedges
- 2 tbsps. chopped capers
- 4 flounder fillets
- Salt and pepper, to taste

1. In the Instant Pot, set in a steamer basket and pour the water into the pot.

2. Sprinkle salt and pepper to the flounder fillets. Sprinkle with dill and chopped capers on top. Add lemon wedges on top for garnish.

3. Place the fillets on the trivet.

4. Lock the lid. Select the Steam mode and cook for 10 minutes at Low Pressure.

5. Once cooking is complete, do a quick pressure release. Carefully open the lid.

6. Serve warm.

Halibut En Papillote

Prep time: 12 mins, Cook time: 10 mins, Servings: 4

- 1 cup water
- 1 cup chopped tomatoes
- 1 thinly sliced shallot
- 4 halibut fillets
- ½ tbsp. grated ginger
- Salt and pepper, to taste

1. In the Instant Pot, set in a steamer basket and pour the water into the pot.

2. Get a large parchment paper and place the fillet in the middle. Season with salt and pepper. Add the grated ginger, tomatoes, and shallots. Fold the parchment paper to create a pouch and crimp the edges.

3. Place the parchment paper containing the fish.

4. Lock the lid. Select the Steam mode and cook for 10 minutes at Low Pressure.

5. Once cooking is complete, do a quick pressure release. Carefully open the lid.

6. Serve warm.

Halibut Stew with Bacon

Prep time: 10 minutes | Cook time: 10 minutes | Serves 4

4 slices bacon, chopped

1 celery, chopped

½ cup chopped shallots

1 teaspoon garlic, smashed

1 pound (454 g) halibut

2 cups fish stock

1 tablespoon coconut oil, softened

¼ teaspoon ground allspice

Sea salt and crushed black peppercorns, to taste

1 cup Cottage cheese, at room temperature

1 cup heavy cream

1. Set the Instant Pot to Sauté. Cook the bacon until crispy.

2. Add the celery, shallots, and garlic and sauté for another 2 minutes, or until the vegetables are just tender.

3. Mix in the halibut, stock, coconut oil, allspice, salt, and black peppercorns. Stir well.

4. Lock the lid. Select the Manual mode and set the cooking time for 7 minutes at Low Pressure.

5. When the timer beeps, perform a natural pressure release for 10 minutes, then release any remaining pressure. Carefully remove the lid.

6. Stir in the cheese and heavy cream. Select the Sauté mode again and let it simmer for a few minutes until heated through.

7. Serve immediately.

Pesto Halibut

Prep time: 12 mins, Cook time: 8 mins, Servings: 4

- 2 tbsps. extra virgin olive oil
- 1 tbsp. freshly squeezed lemon juice
- 1 cup basil leaves
- 2 garlic cloves, minced
- 4 halibut fillets
- ¼ cup water
- Salt and pepper, to taste

1. Place the halibut fish in the Instant Pot. Set aside.

2. In a food processor, pulse the basil, olive oil, garlic, and lemon juice until coarse. Sprinkle salt and pepper for seasoning.

3. Spread pesto sauce over halibut fillets. Add the water.

4. Lock the lid. Select the Manual mode and cook for 8 minutes at Low Pressure.

5. Once cooking is complete, do a quick pressure release. Carefully open the lid.

6. Serve warm.

Herbed Cod Steaks

Prep time: 5 minutes | Cook time: 4 minutes | Serves 4

1½ cups water

2 tablespoons garlic-infused oil

4 cod steaks, 1½-inch thick

Sea salt, to taste

½ teaspoon mixed peppercorns, crushed

2 sprigs thyme

1 sprig rosemary

1 yellow onion, sliced

1. Pour the water into your Instant Pot and insert a trivet.
2. Rub the garlic-infused oil into the cod steaks and season with the salt and crushed peppercorns.
3. Lower the cod steaks onto the trivet, skin-side down. Top with the thyme, rosemary, and onion.
4. Lock the lid. Select the Manual mode and set the cooking time for 4 minutes at High Pressure.
5. When the timer beeps, perform a quick pressure release. Carefully remove the lid.
6. Serve immediately.

Salmon with Honey Sauce

Prep time: 10 minutes | Cook time: 0 minutes | Serves 4

Salmon:

1 cup water

1 pound (454 g) salmon fillets

½ teaspoon salt

¼ teaspoon black pepper

Sauce:

½ cup honey

4 cloves garlic, minced

4 tablespoons soy sauce

2 tablespoons rice vinegar

1 teaspoon sesame seeds

1. Pour the water into the Instant Pot and insert a trivet.
2. Season the salmon fillets with salt and pepper to taste, then place on the trivet.
3. Secure the lid. Select the Manual mode and set the cooking time for 0 minutes at High Pressure.

4. Once cooking is complete, do a natural pressure release for 10 minutes, then release any remaining pressure. Carefully open the lid.
5. Meanwhile, whisk together all the ingredients for the sauce in a small bowl until well mixed.
6. Transfer the fillets to a plate and pour the sauce over them. Serve hot.

Curried Salmon

Prep time: 6 mins, Cook Time: 8 mins, Servings: 4

- 2 cups coconut milk
- 2 tbsps. coconut oil
- 1 onion, chopped
- 1 lb. raw salmon, diced
- 1½ tbsps. minced garlic

1. Press the Sauté button on the Instant Pot and heat the oil.
2. Sauté the garlic and onions until fragrant, about 2 minutes.
3. Add the diced salmon and stir for 1 minute.
4. Pour in the coconut milk.
5. Lock the lid. Select the Manual mode and cook for 4 minutes at Low Pressure.
6. Once cooking is complete, do a quick pressure release. Carefully open the lid.
7. Let the salmon cool for 5 minutes before serving.

Italian Salmon with Lemon Juice

Prep time: 6 mins, Cook Time: 8 mins, Servings: 5

- 1½ lbs. salmon fillets
- 2 tbsps. butter
- 3 tbsps. olive oil
- 1 tbsp. Italian herb seasoning mix
- 3 tbsps. freshly squeezed lemon juice
- Salt and pepper, to taste
- ⅓ cup water

1. Place all ingredients in the Instant Pot and stir well.
2. Lock the lid. Select the Manual mode and set the cooking time for 8 minutes at Low Pressure. Flip the fish halfway through the cooking time.
3. Once cooking is complete, do a quick pressure release. Carefully open the lid.
4. Divide the salmon among plates and serve.

Lemon Pepper Salmon

Prep time: 15 mins, Cook time: 5 mins, Servings: 4

- 1 cup water
- 1 tsp. ground dill
- 1 tsp. ground tarragon
- 1 tsp. ground basil
- 4 salmon fillets
- 2 tbsps. olive oil
- Salt, to taste
- 4 lemon slices
- 1 carrot, sliced
- 1 zucchini, sliced

1. In the Instant Pot, add the water, dill, tarragon, and basil.
2. Place the steamer basket inside.
3. Set in the salmon. Drizzle with a tablespoon of olive oil, pepper and salt. Top with lemon slices.
4. Lock the lid. Select the Steam mode and cook for 3 minutes at Low Pressure.
5. Once cooking is complete, do a quick pressure release. Carefully open the lid.
6. Transfer the fish to a plate and discard the lemon slices.
7. Drizzle the Instant Pot with remaining olive oil. Add the carrot and zucchini to the Instant Pot. Set to Sauté mode, then sauté for 2minutes or until the vegetables are tender.
8. Serve the salmon with the veggies.
9. Garnish with fresh lemon wedges.

Lemony Salmon with Avocados

Prep time: 10 minutes | Cook time: 7 minutes | Serves 2

2 (3-ounce / 85-g) salmon fillets
½ teaspoon salt
¼ teaspoon pepper
1 cup water
⅓ cup mayonnaise
Juice of ½ lemon
2 avocados
½ teaspoon chopped fresh dill

1. Season the salmon fillets on all sides with the salt and pepper. Add the water to the Instant Pot and insert a trivet.
2. Arrange the salmon fillets on the trivet, skin-side down.
3. Secure the lid. Select the Steam mode and set the cooking time for 7 minutes at Low Pressure.
4. Once cooking is complete, do a quick pressure release. Carefully open the lid. Set aside to cool.
5. Mix together the mayonnaise and lemon juice in a large bowl. Cut the avocados in half. Remove the pits and dice the avocados. Add the avocados to the large bowl and gently fold into the mixture.
6. Flake the salmon into bite-sized pieces with a fork and gently fold into the mixture.
7. Serve garnished with the fresh dill.

Tilapia Fillets with Arugula

Prep time: 5 minutes | Cook time: 4 minutes | Serves 4

1 lemon, juiced
1 cup water
1 pound (454 g) tilapia fillets
½ teaspoon cayenne pepper, or more to taste
2 teaspoons butter, melted
Sea salt and ground black pepper, to taste
½ teaspoon dried basil
2 cups arugula

1. Pour the fresh lemon juice and water into your Instant Pot and insert a steamer basket.
2. Brush the fish fillets with the melted butter.
3. Sprinkle with the cayenne pepper, salt, and black pepper. Place the tilapia fillets in the basket. Sprinkle the dried basil on top.
4. Lock the lid. Select the Manual mode and set the cooking time for 4 minutes at Low Pressure.
5. When the timer beeps, perform a quick pressure release. Carefully remove the lid.
6. Serve with the fresh arugula.

Lime Tilapia Fillets

Prep time: 10 minutes | Cook time: 2 minutes | Serves 4

1 cup water

4 tablespoons lime juice

3 tablespoons chili powder

½ teaspoon salt

1 pound (454 g) tilapia fillets

1. Pour the water into Instant Pot and insert a trivet.
2. Whisk together the lime juice, chili powder, and salt in a small bowl until combined. Brush both sides of the tilapia fillets generously with the sauce. Put the tilapia fillets on top of the trivet.
3. Secure the lid. Select the Manual mode and set the cooking time for 2 minutes at High Pressure.
4. Once cooking is complete, do a quick pressure release. Carefully open the lid.
5. Remove the tilapia fillets from the Instant Pot to a plate and serve.

Salmon with Mayo

Prep time: 5 minutes | Cook time: 15 minutes | Serves 4 to 6

½ cup mayonnaise

4 cloves garlic, minced

1 tablespoon lemon juice

1 teaspoon dried basil leaves

2 pounds (907 g) salmon fillets

Salt and ground pepper, to taste

2 tablespoons olive oil

Chopped green onion, for garnish

1. Stir together the mayo, garlic, lemon juice, and basil in a bowl. Set aside.
2. Season the salmon fillets with salt and pepper to taste.
3. Press the Sauté button on the Instant Pot and heat the olive oil.
4. Add the seasoned fillets and brown each side for 5 minutes. Add the mayo mixture to the Instant Pot and coat the fillets. Continue cooking for another 5 minutes, flipping occasionally.

5. Remove from the Instant Pot to a plate and serve garnished with the green onions.

Panko Tilapia

Prep time: 15 minutes | Cook time: 18 minutes | Serves 4

1 pound (454 g) tilapia fillets

1 teaspoon salt

½ teaspoon black pepper

1 cup whole milk

3 large eggs, lightly beaten

½ cup panko bread crumbs

6 tablespoons olive oil, divided

1. Season the tilapia with salt and black pepper. Set aside.
2. Place the milk in a shallow bowl, the beaten eggs in a separate shallow bowl, and the panko in a dish.
3. Press the Sauté button on the Instant Pot and heat 2 tablespoons of olive oil.
4. Dredge the tilapia fillets in the milk, then dip in the eggs, shaking off any excess, and finally coat with the panko.
5. Working in batches, place the coated fillets in the hot oil. Cook each side for 3 minutes until evenly browned. Transfer the fillets to a paper towel-lined plate. Repeat with the remaining 4 tablespoons of olive oil and fillets.
6. Cool for 5 minutes and serve.

Perch Fillets with Red Curry

Prep time: 5 minutes | Cook time: 6 minutes | Serves 4

1 cup water

2 sprigs rosemary

1 large-sized lemon, sliced

1 pound (454 g) perch fillets

1 teaspoon cayenne pepper

Sea salt and ground black pepper, to taste

1 tablespoon red curry paste

1 tablespoons butter

1. Add the water, rosemary, and lemon slices to the Instant Pot and insert a trivet.

2. Season the perch fillets with the cayenne pepper, salt, and black pepper. Spread the red curry paste and butter over the fillets.

3. Arrange the fish fillets on the trivet.

4. Lock the lid. Select the Manual mode and set the cooking time for 6 minutes at Low Pressure.

5. When the timer beeps, perform a quick pressure release. Carefully remove the lid.

6. Serve with your favorite keto sides.

Pesto Salmon with Almonds

Prep time: 5 minutes | Cook time: 12 minutes | Serves 4

1 tablespoon butter

¼ cup sliced almonds

4 (3-ounce / 85-g) salmon fillets

½ cup pesto

¼ teaspoon pepper

½ teaspoon salt

1 cup water

1. Press the Sauté button on the Instant Pot and add the butter and almonds.

2. Sauté for 3 to 5 minutes until they start to soften. Remove and set aside.

3. Brush salmon fillets with pesto and season with salt and pepper.

4. Pour the water into Instant Pot and insert the trivet. Place the salmon fillets on the trivet.

5. Secure the lid. Select the Steam mode and set the cooking time for 7 minutes at High Pressure.

6. Once cooking is complete, do a quick pressure release. Carefully open the lid.

7. Serve the salmon with the almonds sprinkled on top.

Quick Salmon

Prep time: 12 mins, Cook Time: 5 mins, Servings: 4

- 1 cup water
- ¼ cup lemon juice
- 1 tbsp. butter
- ¼ tsp. salt
- 4 boneless salmon fillets
- 1 bunch dill, chopped

1. Place the water in the Instant Pot, add lemon juice, add steamer basket, add salmon inside, season with some salt, sprinkle dill and drizzle melted butter.

2. Lock the lid. Select the Manual mode and cook for 5 minutes at Low Pressure.

3. Once cooking is complete, do a quick pressure release. Carefully open the lid.

4. Divide salmon between plates and serve with a side dish.

Red Curry Halibut

Prep time: 3 mins, Cook time: 10 mins, Servings: 4

- 2 tbsps. chopped cilantro
- 4 skinless halibut fillets
- 3 green curry leaves
- 1 cup chopped tomatoes
- 1 tbsp. freshly squeezed lime juice
- Salt and pepper, to taste

1. Place all ingredients in the Instant Pot. Give a good stir to combine the ingredients.

2. Lock the lid. Select the Manual mode and cook for 10 minutes at Low Pressure.

3. Do a quick pressure release.

Salmon Cakes

Prep time: 15 minutes | Cook time: 9 minutes | Serves 4

½ pound (227 g) cooked salmon, shredded

2 medium green onions, sliced

2 large eggs, lightly beaten

1 cup bread crumbs

½ cup chopped flat leaf parsley

¼ cup soy sauce

1 tablespoon Worcestershire sauce

1 teaspoon salt

½ tablespoon garlic powder

½ teaspoon cayenne pepper

¼ teaspoon celery seed

4 tablespoons olive oil, divided

1. Stir together all the ingredients except the olive oil in a large mixing bowl until combined.

2. Set your Instant Pot to Sauté and heat 2 tablespoons of olive oil.

3. Scoop out golf ball-sized clumps of the salmon mixture and roll them into balls, then flatten to form cakes.

4. Working in batches, arrange the salmon cakes in an even layer in the Instant Pot.

5. Cook each side for 2 minutes until golden brown. Transfer to a paper towel-lined plate. Repeat with the remaining 2 tablespoons of olive oil and salmon cakes.

6. Serve immediately.

Salmon with Basil Pesto

Prep time: 6 mins, Cook Time: 6 mins, Servings: 6

- 3 garlic cloves, minced
- 1½ lbs. salmon fillets
- 2 cups basil leaves
- 2 tbsps. freshly squeezed lemon juice
- ½ cup olive oil
- Salt and pepper, to taste

1. Make the pesto sauce: Put the basil leaves, olive oil, lemon juice, and garlic in a food processor, and pulse until smooth.

2. Season with salt and pepper.

3. Place the salmon fillets in the Instant Pot and add the pesto sauce.

4. Lock the lid. Select the Manual mode and set the cooking time for 6 minutes at Low Pressure.

5. Once cooking is complete, do a quick pressure release. Carefully open the lid.

6. Divide the salmon among six plates and serve.

Salmon with Dill

Prep time: 12 mins, Cook Time: 10 mins, Servings: 2

- 2 tbsps. dill
- ⅓ cup olive oil
- 1 tbsp. fresh lemon juice
- 2 tbsps. butter
- 2 salmon fillets
- 1 cup water
- Salt and pepper, to taste

1. Add the water and steam rack to the Instant Pot.

2. Put the remaining ingredients in a heatproof dish and stir well.

3. Place the dish on the steam rack.

4. Lock the lid. Select the Steam mode and cook for 10 minutes at Low Pressure.

5. Once cooking is complete, do a quick pressure release. Carefully open the lid.

6. Divide the salmon fillets among two serving plates and serve.

Snapper with Spicy Tomato Sauce

Prep time: 5 minutes | Cook time: 5 minutes | Serves 6

2 teaspoons coconut oil, melted

1 teaspoon celery seeds

½ teaspoon fresh grated ginger

½ teaspoon cumin seeds

1 yellow onion, chopped

2 cloves garlic, minced

1½ pounds (680 g) snapper fillets

¾ cup vegetable broth

1 (14-ounce / 113-g) can fire-roasted diced tomatoes

1 bell pepper, sliced

1 jalapeño pepper, minced

Sea salt and ground black pepper, to taste

¼ teaspoon chili flakes

½ teaspoon turmeric powder

1. Set the Instant Pot to Sauté. Add and heat the sesame oil until hot. Sauté the celery seeds, fresh ginger, and cumin seeds.

2. Add the onion and continue to sauté until softened and fragrant.

3. Mix in the minced garlic and continue to cook for 30 seconds. Add the remaining ingredients and stir well.

4. Lock the lid. Select the Manual mode and set the cooking time for 3 minutes at Low Pressure.

5. When the timer beeps, perform a quick pressure release. Carefully remove the lid.

6. Serve warm

Chili-Rubbed Tilapia

Prep time: 6 mins, Cook time: 10 mins, Servings: 4

- 1 cup water
- ½ tsp. garlic powder
- 1 lb. skinless tilapia fillet

- 2 tbsps. extra virgin olive oil
- Salt and pepper, to taste
- 2 tbsps. chili powder

1. Set a trivet in the Instant Pot and pour the water into the pot.
2. Season the tilapia fillets with salt, pepper, chili powder, and garlic powder. Drizzle with olive oil on top.
3. Place in the steamer basket.
4. Lock the lid. Select the Steam mode and cook for 10 minutes at Low Pressure.
5. Once cooking is complete, do a quick pressure release. Carefully open the lid.
6. Serve warm.

Steamed Cod and Veggies

Prep time: 5 minutes | Cook time: 2 to 4 minutes | Serves 2

½ cup water
Kosher salt and freshly ground black pepper, to taste
2 tablespoons freshly squeezed lemon juice, divided
2 tablespoons melted butter
1 garlic clove, minced
1 zucchini or yellow summer squash, cut into thick slices
1 cup cherry tomatoes
1 cup whole Brussels sprouts
2 (6-ounce / 170-g) cod fillets
2 thyme sprigs or ½ teaspoon dried thyme
Hot cooked rice, for serving

1. Pour the water into your Instant Pot and insert a steamer basket.
2. Sprinkle the fish with the salt and pepper. Mix together 1 tablespoon of the lemon juice, the butter, and garlic in a small bowl. Set aside.
3. Add the zucchini, tomatoes, and Brussels sprouts to the basket. Sprinkle with the salt and pepper and drizzle the remaining 1 tablespoon of lemon juice over the top.
4. Place the fish fillets on top of the veggies. Brush with the mixture and then turn the fish and repeat on the other side. Drizzle any remaining mixture all over the veggies. Place the thyme sprigs on top.
5. Lock the lid. Select the Steam mode and set the cooking time for 2 to 4 minutes on High Pressure, depending on the thickness of the fish.

6. Once cooking is complete, use a quick pressure release. Carefully open the lid.
7. Serve the cod and veggies over the cooked rice.

Greek Snapper

Prep time: 6 mins, Cook time: 10 mins, Servings: 4
- 1 cup water
- 12 snapper fillets
- 3 tbsps. olive oil
- 2 tbsps. Greek yogurt
- 1 garlic clove, minced
- Salt and pepper, to taste

1. Set a trivet in the Instant Pot and pour the water into the pot.
2. In a mixing bowl, combine the olive oil, garlic, and Greek yogurt. Sprinkle salt and pepper for seasoning.
3. Apply Greek yogurt mixture to the fish fillets. Place the fillets on the trivet.
4. Lock the lid. Select the Steam mode and cook for 10 minutes at Low Pressure.
5. Once cooking is complete, do a quick pressure release. Carefully open the lid.
6. Serve warm.

Herbed Red Snapper

Prep time: 3 mins, Cook time: 12 mins, Servings: 4
- 1 cup water
- 4 red snapper fillets
- 1½ tsps. chopped fresh herbs
- ¼ tsp. paprika
- 3 tbsps. freshly squeezed lemon juice
- Salt and pepper, to taste

1. Set a trivet in the Instant Pot and pour the water into the pot.
2. Mix all ingredients in a heat-proof dish that will fit in the Instant Pot. Combine to coat the fish with all ingredients.
3. Place the heat-proof dish on the trivet.
4. Lock the lid. Select the Manual mode and cook for 12 minutes at Low Pressure.
5. Once cooking is complete, do a quick pressure release. Carefully open the lid.
6. Serve warm.

Salmon with Lemon Mustard

Prep time: 8 mins, Cook time: 10 mins, Servings: 4

- 1 cup water
- 1 garlic clove, minced
- 4 skinless salmon fillets
- 2 tbsps. Dijon mustard
- Salt and pepper, to taste
- 2 tbsps. freshly squeezed lemon juice

1. Set a trivet in the Instant Pot and pour the water into the pot.
2. In a bowl, mix lemon juice, mustard, and garlic. Sprinkle salt and pepper for seasoning.
3. Top the salmon fillets with the mustard mixture. Place the fish fillets on the trivet.
4. Lock the lid. Select the Steam mode and cook for 10 minutes at Low Pressure.
5. Once cooking is complete, do a quick pressure release. Carefully open the lid.
6. Serve warm.

Teriyaki Salmon

Prep time: 5 minutes | Cook time: 0 minutes | Serves 4

1 pound (454 g) salmon fillets

½ cup packed light brown sugar

½ cup rice vinegar

½ cup soy sauce

1 tablespoon cornstarch

1 teaspoon minced ginger

¼ teaspoon garlic powder

1. Place the salmon fillets into the Instant Pot.
2. Whisk together the remaining ingredients in a small bowl until well combined. Pour the mixture over the salmon fillets, turning to coat.
3. Secure the lid. Select the Manual mode and set the cooking time for 0 minutes at High Pressure.
4. Once cooking is complete, do a natural pressure release for 10 minutes, then release any remaining pressure. Carefully open the lid.
5. Serve hot.

Thai Fish Curry

Prep time: 6 mins, Cook Time: 6 mins, Servings: 6

- 1½ lbs. salmon fillets
- 2 cups fresh coconut milk
- ¼ cup chopped cilantro
- ⅓ cup olive oil
- 2 tbsps. curry powder
- Salt and pepper, to taste

1. In the Instant Pot, add all the ingredients. Give a good stir.
2. Lock the lid. Select the Manual mode and set the cooking time for 6 minutes at Low Pressure.
3. Once cooking is complete, do a quick pressure release. Carefully open the lid. Set warm.

Thyme-Sesame Crusted Halibut

Prep time: 6 mins, Cook time: 8 mins, Servings: 4

- 1 cup water
- 1 tsp. dried thyme leaves
- 1 tbsp. toasted sesame seeds
- 8 oz. halibut, sliced
- Salt and pepper, to taste
- 1 tbsp. freshly squeezed lemon juice

1. Set a trivet in the Instant Pot and pour the water into the pot.
2. Season the halibut with lemon juice, salt, and pepper. Sprinkle with dried thyme leaves and sesame seeds.
3. Place the fish on the trivet.
4. Lock the lid. Select the Steam mode and cook for 8 minutes at Low Pressure.
5. Once cooking is complete, do a quick pressure release. Carefully open the lid.
6. Serve warm.

Tilapia Fish Cakes

Prep time: 15 minutes | Cook time: 15 minutes | Serves 4

½ pound (227 g) cooked tilapia fillets, shredded

1½ cups bread crumbs

2 large eggs, lightly beaten

1 cup peeled and shredded russet potato

2 teaspoons lemon juice

2 tablespoons full-fat sour cream

1 teaspoon salt

¼ teaspoon black pepper

½ teaspoon chili powder

⅛ teaspoon cayenne pepper

4 tablespoons olive oil, divided

1.	Mix together all the ingredients except the olive oil in a large bowl and stir until well incorporated.

2.	Scoop out golf ball-sized clumps of the tilapia mixture and roll them into balls, then flatten to form cakes.

3.	Set your Instant Pot to Sauté and heat 2 tablespoons of olive oil.

4.	Put the tilapia cakes in the Instant Pot in an even layer. You'll need to work in batches to avoid overcrowding.

5.	Sear for 2 minutes per side until golden brown. Transfer to a paper towel-lined plate. Repeat with the remaining 2 tablespoons of olive oil and tilapia cakes.

6.	Serve immediately.

Tilapia with Pineapple Salsa

Prep time: 10 minutes | Cook time: 2 minutes | Serves 4

1 pound (454 g) tilapia fillets

¼ teaspoon salt

⅛ teaspoon black pepper

½ cup pineapple salsa

1 cup water

1.	Put the tilapia fillets in the center of a 1½ piece of aluminum foil. Sprinkle the salt and pepper to season.

2.	Fold the sides of the aluminum foil up to resemble a bowl and pour in the pineapple salsa. Fold foil over top of tilapia fillets and crimp the edges.

3.	Pour the water into the Instant Pot and insert a trivet, then put the foil packet on top of the trivet.

4.	Secure the lid. Select the Manual mode and set the cooking time for 2 minutes at High Pressure.

5.	Once cooking is complete, do a quick pressure release. Carefully open the lid.

6.	Remove the foil packet and carefully open it. Serve the tilapia fillets hot with the salsa as garnish.

Tuna Fillets with Lemon Butter

Prep time: 5 minutes | Cook time: 3 minutes | Serves 4

1 cup water

⅓ cup lemon juice

2 sprigs fresh thyme

2 sprigs fresh parsley

2 sprigs fresh rosemary

1 pound (454 g) tuna fillets

4 cloves garlic, pressed

Sea salt, to taste

¼ teaspoon black pepper, or more to taste

2 tablespoons butter, melted

1 lemon, sliced

1.	Pour the water into your Instant Pot. Add the lemon juice, thyme, parsley, and rosemary and insert a steamer basket.

2.	Put the tuna fillets in the basket. Top with the garlic and season with the salt and black pepper.

3.	Drizzle the melted butter over the fish fillets and place the lemon slices on top.

4.	Lock the lid. Select the Manual mode and set the cooking time for 3 minutes at Low Pressure.

5.	When the timer beeps, perform a quick pressure release. Carefully remove the lid.

6.	Serve immediately.

Tuna Noodle Casserole

Prep time: 5 minutes | Cook time: 4 minutes | Serves 4

3 cups water

28 ounces (794 g) cream of mushroom soup

14 ounces (397 g) canned tuna, drained

20 ounces (567 g) egg noodles

1 cup frozen peas

Salt and ground black pepper, to taste

4 ounces (113 g) grated Cheddar cheese

¼ cup bread crumbs (optional)

1.	Combine the water and mushroom soup in the Instant Pot.

2.	Stir in the tuna, egg noodles, and peas. Season with salt and pepper.

3.	Secure the lid. Select the Manual mode and set the cooking time for 4 minutes at High Pressure.

4.	When the timer beeps, perform a quick pressure release. Carefully remove the lid.

5. Scatter the grated cheese and bread crumbs (if desired) on top. Lock the lid and allow to sit for 5 minutes.

6. Serve warm.

Tuna Salad with Lettuce

Prep time: 12 mins, Cook Time: 10 mins, Servings: 4

- 2 tbsps. olive oil
- ½ lb. tuna, sliced
- 1 tbsp. fresh lemon juice
- 2 eggs
- 1 head lettuce
- Salt and pepper, to taste
- 1 cup water

1. In a large bowl, season the tuna with lemon juice, salt and pepper. Transfer the tuna to a baking dish.

2. Add the eggs, water, and steamer rack to the Instant Pot. Place the baking dish on the steamer rack.

3. Lock the lid. Select the Steam mode and set the cooking time for 10 minutes at Low Pressure.

4. Once cooking is complete, do a quick pressure release. Carefully open the lid.

5. Allow the eggs and tuna to cool. Peel the eggs and slice into wedges. Set aside.

6. Assemble the salad by shredding the lettuce in a salad bowl. Toss in the cooled tuna and eggs.

7. Sprinkle with olive oil, then serve.

Wild Alaskan Cod with Cherry Tomatoes

Prep time: 5 minutes | Cook time: 8 minutes | Serves 2

1 large fillet wild Alaskan Cod

1 cup cherry tomatoes, chopped

Salt and ground black pepper, to taste

2 tablespoons butter

1. Add the tomatoes to your Instant Pot. Top with the cod fillet. Sprinkle with the salt and pepper.

2. Secure the lid. Press the Manual button on your Instant Pot and set the cooking time for 8 minutes on High Pressure.

3. Once the timer goes off, perform a quick pressure release. Carefully remove the lid.

4. Add the butter to the cod fillet. Secure the lid and let stand for 1 minute.

5. Transfer to a serving plate and serve.

CHAPTER 5 POULTRY

Double-Cheesy Drumsticks

Prep time: 3 minutes | Cook time: 23 minutes | Serves 5

1 tablespoon olive oil

5 chicken drumsticks

½ cup chicken stock

¼ cup unsweetened coconut milk

¼ cup dry white wine

2 garlic cloves, minced

1 teaspoon shallot powder

½ teaspoon marjoram

½ teaspoon thyme

6 ounces (170 g) ricotta cheese

4 ounces (113 g) Cheddar cheese

½ teaspoon cayenne pepper

¼ teaspoon ground black pepper

Sea salt, to taste

1. Set your Instant Pot to Sauté and heat the olive oil until sizzling.

2. Add the chicken drumsticks and brown each side for 3 minutes.

3. Stir in the chicken stock, milk, wine, garlic, shallot powder, marjoram, thyme.

4. Lock the lid. Select the Manual mode and set the cooking time for 15 minutes at High Pressure.

5. When the timer beeps, perform a natural pressure release for 10 minutes, then release any remaining pressure. Carefully remove the lid.

6. Shred the chicken with two forks and return to the Instant Pot.

7. Set your Instant Pot to Sauté again and add the remaining ingredients and stir well.

8. Cook for another 2 minutes, or until the cheese is melted. Taste and add more salt, if desired. Serve immediately.

Chicken with Jalapeño

Prep time: 15 mins, Cook Time: 12 mins, Servings: 3

- 1 lb. boneless chicken breast
- 3 jalapeños, sliced
- 8 oz. Cheddar cheese
- ¾ cup sour cream
- 8 oz. cream cheese
- Salt and pepper, to taste
- ½ cup water

1. Add ½ cup water, cream cheese, jalapeños, chicken breast, salt, and pepper to the pot. Stir to combine well.

2. Lock the lid. Select the Manual mode and set the cooking time for 12 minutes at High Pressure.

3. Once cooking is complete, do a natural pressure release for 8 minutes, then release any remaining pressure. Carefully open the lid.

4. Mix in the sour cream and Cheddar cheese, and serve warm!

Chicken Fajita Bowls

Prep time: 5 minutes | Cook time: 10 minutes | Serves 2

1 pound (454 g) boneless, skinless chicken breasts, cut into 1-inch pieces

2 cups chicken broth

1 cup salsa

1 teaspoon paprika

1 teaspoon fine sea salt, or more to taste

1 teaspoon chili powder

½ teaspoon ground cumin

½ teaspoon ground black pepper

1 lime, halved

1. Combine all the ingredients except the lime in the Instant Pot.

2. Lock the lid. Select the Manual mode and set the cooking time for 10 minutes at High Pressure.

3. When the timer beeps, perform a quick pressure release. Carefully remove the lid.

4. Shred the chicken with two forks and return to the Instant Pot. Squeeze the lime juice into the chicken mixture. Taste and add more salt, if needed. Give the mixture a good stir.

5. Ladle the chicken mixture into bowls and serve.

Chicken with Cheese Sauce

Prep time: 5 minutes | Cook time: 10 minutes | Serves 4

1 tablespoon olive oil
1 pound (454 g) chicken fillets
½ teaspoon dried basil
Salt and freshly ground black pepper, to taste
1 cup chicken broth
Cheese Sauce:
3 teaspoons butter, at room temperature
⅓ cup grated Gruyère cheese
⅓ cup Neufchâtel cheese, at room temperature
⅓ cup heavy cream
3 tablespoons unsweetened coconut milk
1 teaspoon shallot powder
½ teaspoon granulated garlic

1. Set your Instant Pot to Sauté and heat the olive oil until sizzling.
2. Add the chicken and sear each side for 3 minutes. Sprinkle with the basil, salt, and black pepper.
3. Pour the broth into the Instant Pot and stir well.
4. Lock the lid. Select the Manual mode and set the cooking time for 6 minutes at High Pressure.
5. When the timer beeps, perform a natural pressure release for 10 minutes, then release any remaining pressure. Carefully remove the lid.
6. Transfer the chicken to a platter and set aside.
7. Clean the Instant Pot. Press the Sauté button and melt the butter.
8. Add the cheeses, heavy cream, milk, shallot powder, and garlic, stirring until everything is heated through.
9. Pour the cheese sauce over the chicken and serve.

Chicken Piccata

Prep time: 5 minutes | Cook time: 25 minutes | Serves 4

4 (6-ounce / 170-g) boneless, skinless chicken breasts
½ teaspoon salt
½ teaspoon garlic powder
¼ teaspoon pepper
2 tablespoons coconut oil
1 cup water
2 cloves garlic, minced

4 tablespoons butter
Juice of 1 lemon
¼ teaspoon xanthan gum

1. Sprinkle the chicken with salt, garlic powder, and pepper.
2. Set your Instant Pot to Sauté and melt the coconut oil.
3. Add the chicken and sear each side for about 5 to 7 minutes until golden brown.
4. Remove the chicken and set aside on a plate.
5. Pour the water into the Instant Pot. Using a wooden spoon, scrape the bottom if necessary, to remove any stuck-on seasoning or meat. Insert the trivet and place the chicken on the trivet.
6. Secure the lid. Select the Manual mode and set the cooking time for 10 minutes at High Pressure.
7. Once cooking is complete, do a natural pressure release for 10 minutes, then release any remaining pressure. Carefully open the lid.
8. Remove the chicken and set aside. Strain the broth from the Instant Pot into a large bowl and return to the pot.
9. Set your Instant Pot to Sauté again and add the remaining ingredients. Cook for at least 5 minutes, stirring frequently, or until the sauce is cooked to your desired thickness.
10. Pour the sauce over the chicken and serve warm.

Chicken and Cranberry Salad

Prep time: 10 minutes | Cook time: 6 to 10 minutes | Serves 2

1 pound (454 g) skinless, boneless chicken breasts
½ cup water
2 teaspoons kosher salt, plus more for seasoning
½ cup mayonnaise
1 celery stalk, diced
2 tablespoons diced red onion
½ cup chopped dried cranberries
¼ cup chopped walnuts
1 tablespoon freshly squeezed lime juice
¼ shredded unpeeled organic green apple
Freshly ground black pepper, to taste

1.   Add the chicken, water, and 2 teaspoons of salt to your Instant Pot.
2.   Lock the lid. Press the Poultry button on the Instant Pot and cook for 6 minutes on High Pressure.
3.   Once cooking is complete, use a natural pressure release for 5 minutes and then release any remaining pressure. Carefully open the lid.
4.   Remove the chicken from the Instant Pot to a cutting board and let sit for 5 to 10 minutes.
5.   Shred the meat, transfer to a bowl, and add ¼ cup of the cooking liquid.
6.   Mix in the mayonnaise and stir until well coated. Add the celery, onion, cranberries, walnuts, lime juice, and apple. Sprinkle with the salt and pepper.
7.   Serve immediately.

Chicken and Spinach Stew

Prep time: 13 mins, Cook time: 10 mins, Servings: 6
- 1 ginger, sliced
- 3 garlic cloves, minced
- 2 cups spinach leaves
- 1 cup chopped tomatoes
- 1 lb. chicken breasts
- 1 cup water
- Salt and pepper, to taste

1.   Press the Sauté button on the Instant Pot and add the chicken and garlic. Stir-fry for 3 minutes until the garlic becomes fragrant.
2.   Add the ginger, tomatoes, spinach, and water. Season with salt and pepper.
3.   Lock the lid. Select the Manual mode and set the cooking time for 6 minutes at High Pressure.
4.   Once cooking is complete, do a natural pressure release for 5 minutes, then release any remaining pressure. Carefully open the lid.
5.   Cool for a few minutes and serve warm.

Chicken Tacos with Cheese Shells

Prep time: 5 minutes | Cook time: 25 minutes | Serves 6
Chicken:
4 (6-ounce / 170-g) boneless, skinless chicken breasts
1 cup chicken broth

1 teaspoon salt
¼ teaspoon pepper
1 tablespoon chili powder
2 teaspoons garlic powder
2 teaspoons cumin
Cheese Shells:
1½ cups shredded whole-milk Mozzarella cheese

1.   Combine all ingredients for the chicken in the Instant Pot.
2.   Secure the lid. Select the Manual mode and set the cooking time for 20 minutes at High Pressure.
3.   Once cooking is complete, do a quick pressure release. Carefully open the lid.
4.   Shred the chicken and serve in bowls or cheese shells.
5.   Make the cheese shells: Heat a nonstick skillet over medium heat.
6.   Sprinkle ¼ cup of Mozzarella cheese in the skillet and fry until golden. Flip and turn off the heat. Allow the cheese to get brown. Fill with chicken and fold. The cheese will harden as it cools. Repeat with the remaining cheese and filling.
7.   Serve warm.

Chicken Verde with Green Chile

Prep time: 5 minutes | Cook time: 15 minutes | Serves 4
3 pounds (1.4 kg) bone-in, skin-on chicken drumsticks and/or thighs
1 (27-ounce / 765-g) can roasted poblano peppers, drained
1 (15-ounce / 425-g) jar salsa verde (green chile salsa)
1 (7-ounce / 198-g) jar chopped green chiles, drained
1 onion, chopped
1 tablespoon chopped jalapeño (optional)
1 tablespoon ground cumin
4 teaspoons minced garlic
1 teaspoon fine sea salt

1.   Mix together all the ingredients in your Instant Pot and stir to combine.
2.   Secure the lid. Press the Manual button and set the cooking time for 15 minutes on High Pressure.
3.   Once the timer goes off, use a quick pressure release. Carefully open the lid.

4. Remove the chicken from the Instant Pot to a plate with tongs. Let cool for 5 minutes.

5. Remove the bones and skin and discard. Shred the chicken with two forks.

6. Transfer the chicken back to the sauce and stir to combine.

7. Serve immediately.

Chicken Wingettes with Cilantro Sauce

Prep time: 5 minutes | Cook time: 6 minutes | Serves 6

12 chicken wingettes

10 fresh cayenne peppers, trimmed and chopped

3 garlic cloves, minced

1½ cups white vinegar

1 teaspoon sea salt

1 teaspoon onion powder

½ teaspoon black pepper

2 tablespoons olive oil

Dipping Sauce:

½ cup sour cream

½ cup mayonnaise

½ cup cilantro, chopped

2 cloves garlic, minced

1 teaspoon smoked paprika

1. In a large bowl, toss the chicken wingettes, cayenne peppers, garlic, white vinegar, salt, onion powder, and black pepper. Cover and marinate for 1 hour in the refrigerator.

2. When ready, transfer the chicken wingettes to the Instant Pot, along with the marinade and olive oil.

3. Lock the lid. Select the Manual mode and set the cooking time for 6 minutes at High Pressure.

4. Meanwhile, thoroughly combine all the sauce ingredients in a mixing bowl.

5. When the timer beeps, perform a quick pressure release. Carefully remove the lid.

6. Serve the chicken warm alongside the dipping sauce.

Super Garlicky Chicken

Prep time: 5 minutes | Cook time: 20 minutes | Serves 6

1 tablespoon butter

1 tablespoon olive oil

2 chicken breasts, bone and skin not removed

4 chicken thighs, bone and skin not removed

Salt and pepper, to taste

40 cloves of garlic, peeled and sliced

2 sprigs of thyme

¼ cup chicken broth

¼ cup dry white wine

Parsley, for garnish

1. Set your Instant Pot to Sauté. Add the butter and oil.

2. Fold in the chicken pieces and stir well. Sprinkle with the salt and pepper.

3. Mix in the garlic cloves and sauté for an additional 5 minutes until fragrant.

4. Add the thyme, chicken broth, and white wine. Stir well.

5. Secure the lid. Select the Manual mode and set the cooking time for 15 minutes on High Pressure.

6. Once cooking is complete, use a quick pressure release. Carefully open the lid.

7. Transfer to a serving dish and serve garnished with parsley.

Chicken with Artichokes and Bacon

Prep time: 10 mins, Cook Time: 25 mins, Servings:4

- 2 chicken breasts, skinless, boneless, and halved
- 2 cups canned artichokes, drained, and chopped
- 1 cup bacon, cooked and crumbled
- 1 cup water
- 2 tbsps. tomato paste
- 1 tbsp. chives, chopped
- Salt, to taste

1. Mix all the ingredients in your Instant Pot until well combined.

2. Lock the lid. Select the Poultry mode and set the cooking time for 25 minutes at High Pressure.

3. Once cooking is complete, do a natural pressure release for 10 minutes, then release any remaining pressure. Carefully open the lid.

4. Remove from the pot to a large plate and serve.

Chili Chicken Zoodles

Prep time: 10 minutes | Cook time: 20 minutes | Serves 4

2 chicken breasts, skinless, boneless and halved

1½ cups chicken stock

3 celery stalks, chopped

1 tablespoon tomato sauce

1 teaspoon chili powder

A pinch of salt and black pepper

2 zucchinis, spiralized

1 tablespoon chopped cilantro

1. Mix together all the ingredients except the zucchini noodles and cilantro in the Instant Pot.
2. Secure the lid. Select the Manual mode and set the cooking time for 15 minutes at High Pressure.
3. Once cooking is complete, do a natural pressure release for 10 minutes, then release any remaining pressure. Carefully open the lid.
4. Set your Instant Pot to Sauté and add the zucchini noodles. Cook for about 5 minutes, stirring often, or until softened.
5. Sprinkle the cilantro on top for garnish before serving.

Lime-Chili Chicken

Prep time: 12 mins, Cook time: 6 mins, Servings:5

- 6 garlic cloves, minced
- 1 tbsp. chili powder
- 1 tsp. cumin
- 1 lb. skinless and boneless chicken breasts
- 1 ½ limes, juiced
- 1 cup water

1. In the Instant Pot, add the chicken breasts, garlic, chili powder, cumin, lime juice, salt, pepper, and water.
2. Lock the lid. Select the Manual mode and cook for 6 minutes at High Pressure.
3. Once cooking is complete, do a natural pressure release for 5 minutes, then release any remaining pressure. Carefully open the lid.
4. Cool for 5 minutes and serve warm.

Chinese Steamed Chicken

Prep time: 6 mins, Coo time: 10 mins, Servings: 6

- 1 tsp. grated ginger
- 1½ lbs. chicken thighs
- 1 tbsp. five-spice powder
- ¼ cup soy sauce
- 3 tbsps. sesame oil
- 1 cup water
- Salt and pepper, to taste

1. In the Instant Pot, stir in all the ingredients.
2. Lock the lid. Select the Poultry mode and set the cooking time for 10 minutes at High Pressure.
3. Once cooking is complete, do a natural pressure release for 7 minutes, then release any remaining pressure. Carefully open the lid.
4. Serve the chicken thighs while warm.

Chipotle Chicken Fajita

Prep time: 15 minutes | Cook time: 10 minutes | Serves 2

1 tablespoon oil

½ green bell pepper, sliced

¼ red onion, sliced

2 skinless, boneless chicken breasts

½ cup water

2 canned chipotle chiles in adobo sauce, deseeded and minced

Kosher salt, to taste

3 tablespoons mayonnaise

¼ cup sour cream

½ tablespoon freshly squeezed lime juice

Freshly ground black pepper, to taste

1. Set your Instant Pot to Sauté and heat the oil until it shimmers.
2. Add the bell pepper and onion and sauté for 3 to 4 minutes until tender.
3. Remove from the Instant Pot to a small bowl and set aside to cool.
4. Add the chicken breasts, water, and a few teaspoons of adobo sauce to the pot and season with salt to taste.
5. Lock the lid. Select the Poultry mode and set the cooking time for 6 minutes at High Pressure.

6. Once cooking is complete, do a natural pressure release for 5 minutes, then release any remaining pressure. Carefully open the lid.

7. Remove the chicken from the pot to a cutting board and allow to cool for 10 minutes. Slice the chicken breasts into cubes and place in a medium bowl.

8. Add the cooked bell pepper and onion, mayo, sour cream, chipotle chiles, lime juice, salt, and pepper to the bowl of chicken and toss to coat. Serve immediately.

Citrus Chicken Tacos

Prep time: 5 minutes | Cook time: 20 minutes | Serves 12

¼ cup olive oil

12 chicken breasts, skin and bones removed

8 cloves of garlic, minced

⅔ cup orange juice, freshly squeezed

⅔ cup lime juice, freshly squeezed

2 tablespoons ground cumin

1 tablespoon dried oregano

1 tablespoon orange peel

Salt and pepper, to taste

¼ cup cilantro, chopped

1. Set your Instant Pot to Sauté. Add and heat the oil.

2. Add the chicken breasts and garlic. Cook until the chicken pieces are lightly browned.

3. Add the orange juice, lime juice, cumin, oregano, orange peel, salt, and pepper. Stir well.

4. Secure the lid. Select the Poultry mode and cook for 15 minutes on High Pressure.

5. Once cooking is complete, do a quick pressure release. Carefully remove the lid.

6. Serve garnished with the cilantro.

Chicken Breasts with Cream Cheese

Prep time: 5 minutes | Cook time: 15 minutes | Serves 2

½ pound (227 g) boneless, skinless chicken breasts

2 ounces (57 g) cream cheese, softened

½ cup grass-fed bone broth

¼ cup tablespoons keto-friendly ranch dressing

½ cup shredded full-fat Cheddar cheese

3 slices bacon, cooked and chopped into small pieces

1. Combine all the ingredients except the Cheddar cheese and bacon in the Instant Pot.

2. Secure the lid. Select the Manual mode and set the cooking time for 15 minutes at High Pressure.

3. Once cooking is complete, do a quick pressure release. Carefully open the lid.

4. Add the Cheddar cheese and bacon and stir well, then serve.

Crack Chicken with Bacon

Prep time: 5 minutes | Cook time: 15 minutes | Serves 2

½ cup grass-fed bone broth

½ pound (227 g) boneless, skinless chicken breasts

2 ounces (57 g) cream cheese, softened

¼ cup tablespoons keto-friendly ranch dressing

3 slices bacon, cooked, chopped into small pieces

½ cup shredded full-fat Cheddar cheese

1. Add the bone broth, chicken, cream cheese, and ranch dressing to your Instant Pot and stir to combine.

2. Secure the lid. Press the Manual button and set the cooking time for 15 minutes on High Pressure.

3. When the timer goes off, do a quick pressure release. Carefully open the lid.

4. Add the bacon and cheese and stir until the cheese has melted.

5. Serve.

Chicken Cordon Bleu

Prep time: 12 minutes | Cook time: 15 minutes | Serves 6

4 boneless, skinless chicken breast halves, butterflied

4 (1-ounce / 28-g) slices Swiss cheese

8 (1-ounce / 28-g) slices ham

1 cup water

Chopped fresh flat-leaf parsley, for garnish

Sauce:

1½ ounces (43 g) cream cheese (3 tablespoons)

¼ cup chicken broth

1 tablespoon unsalted butter

¼ teaspoon ground black pepper

¼ teaspoon fine sea salt

1. Lay the chicken breast halves on a clean work surface. Top each with a slice of Swiss cheese and 2 slices of ham. Roll the chicken around the ham and cheese, then secure with toothpicks. Set aside.

2. Whisk together all the ingredients for the sauce in a small saucepan over medium heat, stirring until the cream cheese melts and the sauce is smooth.

3. Place the chicken rolls, seam-side down, in a casserole dish. Pour half of the sauce over the chicken rolls. Set the remaining sauce aside.

4. Pour the water into the Instant Pot and insert the trivet. Place the dish on the trivet.

5. Lock the lid. Select the Manual mode and set the cooking time for 15 minutes at High Pressure.

6. When the timer beeps, perform a natural pressure release for 10 minutes, then release any remaining pressure. Carefully remove the lid.

7. Remove the chicken rolls from the Instant Pot to a plate. Pour the remaining sauce over them and serve garnished with the parsley.

Chicken with Cilantro

Prep time: 5 minutes | Cook time: 25 minutes | Serves 4

2 chicken breasts, skinless, boneless and halved

1 cup tomato sauce

1 cup plain Greek yogurt

¾ cup coconut cream

¼ cup chopped cilantro

2 teaspoons garam masala

2 teaspoons ground cumin

A pinch of salt and black pepper

1. Thoroughly combine all the ingredients in the Instant Pot.

2. Lock the lid. Select the Poultry mode and set the cooking time for 25 minutes at High Pressure.

3. Once cooking is complete, do a natural pressure release for 5 minutes, then release any remaining pressure. Carefully open the lid.

4. Transfer the chicken breasts to a plate and serve.

Creamy Chicken with Mushrooms

Prep time: 12 mins, Cook time: 13 mins, Servings: 6

- 4 garlic cloves, minced
- 1 onion, chopped
- 1 cup mushrooms, sliced
- 6 boneless chicken breasts, halved
- ½ cup coconut milk
- ½ cup water

1. Press the Sauté button on the Instant Pot and stir in the chicken breasts.

2. Fold in the onions and garlic and sauté for at least 3 minutes until tender. Season with salt and pepper. Add the remaining ingredients to the Instant Pot and whisk well.

3. Lock the lid. Select the Poultry mode and cook for 8 minutes at High Pressure.

4. Once cooking is complete, do a natural pressure release for 5 minutes, then release any remaining pressure. Carefully open the lid.

5. Allow to cool for 5 minutes before serving.

Crispy Wings

Prep time: 15 mins, Cook time: 15 mins, Servings: 8

- 1 tbsp. paprika
- 1 tsp. rosemary leaves
- Salt and pepper, to taste
- 2 lbs. chicken wings
- 1 cup water

1. Put all the ingredients in the Instant Pot and stir well.

2. Lock the lid. Select the Manual mode and set the cooking time for 15 minutes at High Pressure.

3. Once cooking is complete, do a natural pressure release for 10 minutes, then release any remaining pressure. Carefully open the lid.

4. Transfer to a plate and serve.

Crispy Herbed Chicken

Prep time: 10 mins, Cook Time: 30 mins, Servings: 2 to 3

- 2 tbsps. butter, softened
- ½ head of garlic, crushed
- 1 thyme sprig, crushed
- 1 rosemary sprig, crushed

- ½ tbsp. paprika
- Salt and ground black pepper, to taste
- 1½ lbs. whole chicken, patted dry
- 2 cups water

1. Mix together the butter, garlic, thyme, rosemary, paprika, salt, and pepper in a shallow dish, and stir to incorporate.
2. Slather the butter mixture all over the chicken until well coated. Add the water and chicken to the Instant Pot.
3. Lock the lid. Select the Manual mode and cook for 20 minutes at High Pressure.
4. Once cooking is complete, do a natural pressure release for 10 minutes, then release any remaining pressure. Carefully open the lid.
5. Remove the chicken from the pot and place it under the broiler for 10 minutes, or until the skin is just lightly crisped. Serve warm.

Curried Chicken Legs with Mustard

Prep time: 10 minutes | Cook time: 20 minutes | Serves 5

5 chicken legs, boneless, skin-on
2 garlic cloves, halved
Sea salt, to taste
½ teaspoon smoked paprika
¼ teaspoon ground black pepper
2 teaspoons olive oil
1 tablespoon yellow mustard
1 teaspoon curry paste
4 strips pancetta, chopped
1 shallot, peeled and chopped
1 cup vegetable broth

1. Rub the chicken legs with the garlic halves. Sprinkle with salt, paprika, and black pepper.
2. Set your Instant Pot to Sauté and heat the olive oil.
3. Add the chicken legs and brown for 4 to 5 minutes. Add a splash of chicken broth to deglaze the bottom of the pot.
4. Spread the chicken legs with mustard and curry paste.
5. Add the pancetta strips, shallot, and remaining vegetable broth to the Instant Pot.

6. Lock the lid. Select the Manual mode and set the cooking time for 14 minutes at High Pressure.
7. When the timer beeps, perform a natural pressure release for 10 minutes, then release any remaining pressure. Carefully remove the lid.
8. Serve warm.

Asian Chicken

Prep time: 12 mins, Cook time: 10 mins, Servings: 5
- 3 minced garlic cloves
- ¼ cup chicken broth
- 1½ lbs. boneless chicken breasts
- 3 tbsps. soy sauce
- 1 tbsp. ginger slices

1. Place all ingredients in the Instant Pot. Give a good stir.
2. Lock the lid. Press the Poultry button and set the cooking time for 10 minutes.
3. Once cooking is complete, do a natural pressure release for 8 minutes, then release any remaining pressure. Carefully open the lid.
4. Garnish with chopped scallions and drizzle with sesame oil, if desired.

Kung Pao Chicken

Prep time: 5 minutes | Cook time: 17 minutes | Serves 5
2 tablespoons coconut oil
1 pound (454 g) boneless, skinless chicken breasts, cubed
1 cup cashews, chopped
6 tablespoons hot sauce
½ teaspoon chili powder
½ teaspoon finely grated ginger
½ teaspoon kosher salt
½ teaspoon freshly ground black pepper

1. Set the Instant Pot to Sauté and melt the coconut oil.
2. Add the remaining ingredients to the Instant Pot and mix well.
3. Secure the lid. Select the Manual mode and set the cooking time for 17 minutes at High Pressure.
4. Once cooking is complete, do a quick pressure release. Carefully open the lid.
5. Serve warm.

Chicken and Eggplant Sauté

Prep time: 6 mins, Cook time: 10 mins, Servings: 6

- 3 eggplants, sliced
- 1 tbsp. coconut oil
- 1 tsp. red pepper flakes
- 1 lb. ground chicken
- Salt and pepper, to taste

1. Press the Sauté button on the Instant Pot and heat the coconut oil.
2. Stir in the ground chicken and cook for 3 minutes until lightly golden.
3. Add the remaining ingredients and stir to combine.
4. Lock the lid. Select the Poultry mode and set the cooking time for 6 minutes at High Pressure.
5. Once cooking is complete, do a quick pressure release. Carefully open the lid.
6. Transfer to a large plate and serve warm.

Fennel Chicken

Prep time: 10 mins, Cook Time: 25 mins, Servings: 4

- 2 tbsps. olive oil
- 2 tbsps. grated ginger
- 2 chicken breasts, skinless, boneless and halved
- 1 cup chicken stock
- 2 fennel bulbs, sliced
- 1 tbsp. basil, chopped
- A pinch of salt and black pepper

1. Set your Instant Pot to Sauté and heat the olive oil. Cook the ginger and chicken breasts for 5 minutes until evenly browned.
2. Add the remaining ingredients to the pot and mix well.
3. Lock the lid. Select the Poultry mode and cook for 20 minutes at High Pressure.
4. Once cooking is complete, do a natural pressure release for 10 minutes, then release any remaining pressure. Carefully open the lid.
5. Allow the chicken cool for 5 minutes before serving.

Filipino Chicken Adobo

Prep time: 3 mins, Cook Time: 30 mins, Servings:4

Ingredients
- 4 chicken legs
- ⅓ cup soy sauce
- ¼ cup white vinegar
- ¼ cup sugar
- 5 cloves garlic, crushed
- 2 bay leaves
- 1 onion, chopped
- Salt and pepper, to taste

1. Add all the ingredients to your Instant Pot and stir to combine well.
2. Lock the lid. Select the Poultry mode and cook for 30 minutes at High Pressure.
3. Once cooking is complete, do a natural pressure release for 10 minutes, then release any remaining pressure. Carefully open the lid.
4. Divide the chicken legs among four plates and serve warm.

Garlic Chicken

Prep time: 10 minutes | Cook time: 20 minutes | Serves 4

2 chicken breasts, skinless, boneless and halved

1 cup tomato sauce

¼ cup sweet chili sauce

¼ cup chicken stock

4 garlic cloves, minced

1 tablespoon chopped basil

1. Combine all the ingredients in the Instant Pot.
2. Secure the lid. Select the Poultry mode and set the cooking time for 20 minutes at High Pressure.
3. Once cooking is complete, do a natural pressure release for 10 minutes, then release any remaining pressure. Carefully open the lid.
4. Divide the chicken breasts among four plates and serve.

Ginger Chicken Congee

Prep time: 12 mins, Cook Time: 25 mins, Servings: 4

- 2 cups rice
- 8 medium chicken breasts
- 4 cups water
- 4-inch minced ginger piece
- 1 chicken stock cube
- Salt and pepper, to taste

1. Add the rice, water, chicken breasts, chicken stock, and ginger to the Instant Pot. Season with salt and pepper.
2. Lock the lid. Select the Poultry mode and set the cooking time for 25 minutes at High Pressure.
3. Once cooking is complete, do a natural pressure release for 10 minutes, then release any remaining pressure. Carefully open the lid. Serve warm.

Honey-Glazed Chicken with Sesame

Prep time: 5 minutes | Cook time: 25 minutes | Serves 6

1 tablespoon olive oil
2 cloves garlic, minced
½ cup diced onions
4 large boneless, skinless chicken breasts
Salt and pepper, to taste
½ cup soy sauce
½ cup honey
¼ cup ketchup
2 teaspoons sesame oil
¼ teaspoon red pepper flakes
2 green onions, chopped
1 tablespoon sesame seeds, toasted

1. Press the Sauté button on the Instant Pot and heat the olive oil.
2. Add the garlic and onions and sauté for about 3 minutes until fragrant.
3. Add the chicken breasts and sprinkle with the salt and pepper. Brown each side for 3 minutes.
4. Stir in the soy sauce, honey, ketchup, sesame oil, and red pepper flakes.
5. Secure the lid. Select the Poultry mode and set the cooking time for 20 minutes at High Pressure.

6. Once cooking is complete, do a natural pressure release for 10 minutes, then release any remaining pressure. Carefully open the lid.
7. Sprinkle the onions and sesame seeds on top for garnish before serving.

Huli Huli Chicken

Prep time: 5 minutes | Cook time: 10 minutes | Serves 8

1 cup crushed pineapple, drained
⅓ cup reduced-sodium soy sauce
¾ cup ketchup
3 tablespoons lime juice
3 tablespoons packed brown sugar
1 garlic clove, minced
8 boneless, skinless chicken thighs, about 2 pounds (907 g)
Hot cooked rice, for serving

1. Mix together the pineapple, soy sauce, ketchup, lime juice, sugar, and clove in a mixing bowl.
2. Add the chicken to your Instant Pot and place the mixture on top.
3. Secure the lid. Press the Manual button on the Instant Pot and set the cooking time for 10 minutes at High Pressure.
4. Once cooking is complete, use a natural pressure release for 5 minutes and then release any remaining pressure. Carefully open the lid.
5. Serve with the cooked rice.

Indian Butter Chicken

Prep time: 10 minutes | Cook time: 15 minutes | Serves 4

3 tablespoons butter or ghee, at room temperature, divided
1 medium yellow onion, halved and sliced through the root end
1 (10-ounce / 284-g) can Ro-Tel tomatoes with green chilies, with juice
2 tablespoons mild Indian curry paste
1½ pounds (680 g) boneless, skinless chicken thighs, fat trimmed, cut into 2- to 3-inch pieces
2 tablespoons all-purpose flour

Salt and freshly ground black pepper, to taste

1.   Add 1 tablespoon of the butter in the Instant Pot and select the Sauté mode. Add the onion and sauté for 6 minutes until browned.

2.   Stir in the tomatoes and scrape any browned bits from the pot. Add the curry paste and stir well. Fold in the chicken and stir to coat.

3.   Secure the lid. Press the Manual button on the Instant Pot and cook for 8 minutes on High Pressure.

4.   Once cooking is complete, use a quick pressure release.

5.   Combine the remaining 2 tablespoons of butter and the flour in a small bowl and stir until smooth.

6.   Select the Sauté mode. Add the flour mixture to the chicken in two additions, stirring between additions. Sauté for 1 minute, or until the sauce is thickened.

7.   Sprinkle with the salt and pepper and serve.

Instant Pot Ranch Chicken

Prep time: 5 minutes | Cook time: 20 minutes | Serves 6

1 teaspoon salt

½ teaspoon garlic powder

¼ teaspoon pepper

¼ teaspoon dried oregano

3 (6-ounce / 170-g) skinless chicken breasts

1 stick butter

8 ounces (227 g) cream cheese

1 dry ranch packet

1 cup chicken broth

1.   In a small bowl, combine the salt, garlic powder, pepper, and oregano. Rub this mixture over both sides of chicken breasts.

2.   Place the chicken breasts into the Instant Pot, along with the butter, cream cheese, ranch seasoning, and chicken broth.

3.   Secure the lid. Select the Manual mode and set the cooking time for 20 minutes at High Pressure.

4.   Once cooking is complete, do a natural pressure release for 10 minutes, then release any remaining pressure. Carefully open the lid.

5.   Remove the chicken and shred with two forks, then return to the Instant Pot. Use a rubber spatula to stir and serve on a plate.

Jamaican Curry Chicken Drumsticks

Prep time: 5 minutes | Cook time: 20 minutes | Serves 4

1½ pounds (680 g) chicken drumsticks

1 tablespoon Jamaican curry powder

1 teaspoon salt

1 cup chicken broth

½ medium onion, diced

½ teaspoon dried thyme

1.   Sprinkle the salt and curry powder over the chicken drumsticks.

2.   Place the chicken drumsticks into the Instant Pot, along with the remaining ingredients.

3.   Secure the lid. Select the Manual mode and set the cooking time for 20 minutes at High Pressure.

4.   Once cooking is complete, do a quick pressure release. Carefully open the lid. Serve warm.

Bruschetta Chicken

Prep time: 5 minutes | Cook time: 20 minutes | Serves 2

½ cup filtered water

2 boneless, skinless chicken breasts

1 (14-ounce / 397-g) can sugar-free or low-sugar crushed tomatoes

¼ teaspoon dried basil

½ cup shredded full-fat Cheddar cheese

¼ cup heavy whipping cream

1.   Add the filtered water, chicken breasts, tomatoes, and basil to your Instant Pot.

2.   Lock the lid. Press the Manual button and set the cooking time for 20 minutes on High Pressure.

3.   Once cooking is complete, use a quick pressure release. Carefully open the lid.

4.   Fold in the cheese and cream and stir until the cheese is melted.

5.   Serve immediately.

Paprika Chicken with Tomatoes

Prep time: 10 mins, Cook Time: 20 mins, Servings:4

- 1 tbsp. avocado oil
- 1½ lbs. chicken breast, skinless, boneless, and cubed
- 1 cup tomatoes, cubed
- 1 cup chicken stock

- 1 tbsp. smoked paprika
- 1 tsp. cayenne pepper
- A pinch of salt and black pepper

1. Set your Instant Pot to Sauté and heat the oil. Cook the cubed chicken in the hot oil for 2 to 3 minutes until lightly browned.
2. Add the remaining ingredients to the pot and stir well.
3. Lock the lid. Select the Poultry mode and set the cooking time for 18 minutes at High Pressure.
4. Once cooking is complete, do a natural pressure release for 10 minutes, then release any remaining pressure. Carefully open the lid.
5. Serve the chicken and tomatoes in bowls while warm.

Parmesan Drumsticks

Prep time: 5 minutes | Cook time: 25 minutes | Serves 4
2 pounds (907 g) chicken drumsticks (about 8 pieces)
1 teaspoon salt
1 teaspoon dried parsley
½ teaspoon garlic powder
½ teaspoon dried oregano
¼ teaspoon pepper
1 cup water
1 stick butter
2 ounces (57 g) cream cheese, softened
½ cup grated Parmesan cheese
½ cup chicken broth
¼ cup heavy cream
⅛ teaspoon pepper

1. Sprinkle the salt, parsley, garlic powder, oregano, and pepper evenly over the chicken drumsticks.
2. Pour the water into the Instant Pot and insert the trivet. Arrange the drumsticks on the trivet.
3. Secure the lid. Select the Manual mode and set the cooking time for 15 minutes at High Pressure.
4. Once cooking is complete, do a quick pressure release. Carefully open the lid.
5. Transfer the drumsticks to a foil-lined baking sheet and broil each side for 3 to 5 minutes, or until the skin begins to crisp.

6. Meanwhile, pour the water out of the Instant Pot. Set your Instant Pot to Sauté and melt the butter.
7. Add the remaining ingredients to the Instant Pot and whisk to combine. Pour the sauce over the drumsticks and serve warm.

Prosciutto-Wrapped Chicken

Prep time: 5 minutes | Cook time: 15 minutes | Serves 5
1½ cups water
5 chicken breast halves, butterflied
2 garlic cloves, halved
1 teaspoon marjoram
Sea salt, to taste
½ teaspoon red pepper flakes
¼ teaspoon ground black pepper, or more to taste
10 strips prosciutto

1. Pour the water into the Instant Pot and insert the trivet.
2. Rub the chicken breast halves with garlic. Sprinkle with marjoram, salt, red pepper flakes, and black pepper. Wrap each chicken breast into 2 prosciutto strips and secure with toothpicks. Put the chicken on the trivet.
3. Lock the lid. Select the Poultry mode and set the cooking time for 15 minutes at High Pressure.
4. When the timer beeps, perform a natural pressure release for 10 minutes, then release any remaining pressure. Carefully remove the lid.
5. Remove the toothpicks and serve warm.

Salsa Chicken Legs

Prep time: 5 minutes | Cook time: 16 minutes | Serves 5
5 chicken legs, skinless and boneless
½ teaspoon sea salt
Salsa Sauce:
1 cup puréed tomatoes
1 cup onion, chopped
1 jalapeño, chopped
2 bell peppers, deveined and chopped
2 tablespoons minced fresh cilantro
3 teaspoons lime juice
1 teaspoon granulated garlic

1. Press the Sauté button to heat your Instant Pot.

2.   Add the chicken legs and sear each side for 2 to 3 minutes until evenly browned. Season with sea salt.

3.   Thoroughly combine all the ingredients for the salsa sauce in a mixing bowl. Spoon the salsa mixture evenly over the browned chicken legs.

4.   Lock the lid. Select the Manual mode and set the cooking time for 10 minutes at High Pressure.

5.   When the timer beeps, perform a natural pressure release for 10 minutes, then release any remaining pressure. Carefully remove the lid. Serve warm.

Sesame Chicken

Prep time: 6 mins, Cook time: 25 mins, Servings: 12
- 1½ cup soy sauce
- 1 bay leaf
- 2 packets dried star anise flowers
- 5 lbs. chicken breasts or thighs
- 2 tbsps. toasted sesame seeds
- 2 cups water

1.   Place the chicken breasts, soy sauce, star anise flowers, and bay leaf into the Instant Pot.

2.   Lock the lid. Select the Manual mode and set the cooking time for 25 minutes at High Pressure.

3.   Once cooking is complete, do a natural pressure release for 15 minutes, then release any remaining pressure. Carefully open the lid.

4.   Allow the chicken breasts cool for 5 minutes and serve.

Shredded Chicken

Prep time: 5 minutes | Cook time: 14 minutes | Serves 4
½ teaspoon salt
½ teaspoon pepper
½ teaspoon dried oregano
½ teaspoon dried basil
½ teaspoon garlic powder
2 (6-ounce / 170-g) boneless, skinless chicken breasts
1 tablespoon coconut oil
1 cup water

1.   In a small bowl, combine the salt, pepper, oregano, basil, and garlic powder. Rub this mix over both sides of the chicken.

2.   Set your Instant Pot to Sauté and heat the coconut oil until sizzling.

3.   Add the chicken and sear for 3 to 4 minutes until golden on both sides.

4.   Remove the chicken and set aside.

5.   Pour the water into the Instant Pot and use a wooden spoon or rubber spatula to make sure no seasoning is stuck to bottom of pot.

6.   Add the trivet to the Instant Pot and place the chicken on top.

7.   Secure the lid. Select the Manual mode and set the cooking time for 10 minutes at High Pressure.

8.   Once cooking is complete, do a natural pressure release for 5 minutes, then release any remaining pressure. Carefully open the lid.

9.   Remove the chicken and shred, then serve.

Smoky Chicken

Prep time: 5mins, Cook time: 15 mins, Servings: 6
- 2 tbsps. smoked paprika
- 2 lbs. chicken breasts
- Salt and pepper, to taste
- 1 tbsp. olive oil
- ½ cup water

1.   Press the Sauté button on the Instant Pot and heat the olive oil.

2.   Stir in the chicken breasts and smoked paprika and cook for 3 minutes until lightly golden.

3.   Season with salt and pepper and add ½ cup water.

4.   Lock the lid. Select the Manual mode and cook for 12 minutes at High Pressure.

5.   Once cooking is complete, do a natural pressure release for 8 minutes, then release any remaining pressure. Carefully open the lid.

6.   Garnish with cilantro or scallions, if desired.

Spiced Chicken Drumsticks

Prep time: 6 mins, Cook time: 15 mins, Servings: 10 to 12
- ¼ tsp. dried thyme
- 1½ tbsps. paprika
- Salt and pepper, to taste

- ½ tsp. onion powder
- 12 chicken drumsticks
- 2 cups water

1. On a clean work surface, rub the chicken drumsticks generously with the spices. Season with salt and pepper.
2. Transfer the chicken to the Instant Pot and add the water.
3. Lock the lid. Select the Poultry mode and cook for 15 minutes at High Pressure.
4. Once cooking is complete, do a natural pressure release for 8 minutes, then release any remaining pressure. Carefully open the lid.
5. Remove from the pot to a plate and serve.

Spicy Chicken with Smoked Sausage

Prep time: 35 minutes | Cook time: 15 minutes | Serves 11

1 (6-ounce / 170-g) can tomato paste
1 (14½-ounce / 411-g) can diced tomatoes, undrained
1 (14½-ounce / 411-g) can beef broth or chicken broth
2 medium green peppers, chopped
1 medium onion, chopped
5 garlic cloves, minced
3 celery ribs, chopped
3 teaspoons dried parsley flakes
2 teaspoons dried basil
1½ teaspoons dried oregano
½ teaspoon hot pepper sauce
1¼ teaspoons salt
½ teaspoon cayenne pepper
1 pound (454 g) smoked sausage, halved and cut into ¼-inch slices
1 pound (454 g) boneless, skinless chicken breasts, cut into 1-inch cubes
½ pound (227 g) uncooked shrimp, peeled and deveined
Hot cooked rice, for serving

1. Mix together the tomato paste, tomatoes, and broth in your Instant Pot. Stir in the green peppers, onion, garlic, celery, and seasonings. Fold in the sausage and chicken.
2. Secure the lid. Press the Manual button and set the cooking time for 8 minutes on High Pressure.
3. Once the timer goes off, do a quick pressure release. Carefully open the lid.
4. Set the Instant Pot to sauté. Add the shrimp and stir well. Cook for another 5 minutes, or until the shrimp turn pink, stirring occasionally.
5. Serve over the cooked rice.

Spinach and Feta Stuffed Chicken

Prep time: 10 minutes | Cook time: 25 minutes | Serves 4

½ cup frozen spinach
⅓ cup crumbled feta cheese
1¼ teaspoons salt, divided
4 (6-ounce / 170-g) boneless, skinless chicken breasts, butterflied
¼ teaspoon pepper
¼ teaspoon dried oregano
¼ teaspoon dried parsley
¼ teaspoon garlic powder
2 tablespoons coconut oil
1 cup water

1. Combine the spinach, feta cheese, and ¼ teaspoon of salt in a medium bowl. Divide the mixture evenly and spoon onto the chicken breasts.
2. Close the chicken breasts and secure with toothpicks or butcher's string. Sprinkle the chicken with the remaining 1 teaspoon of salt, pepper, oregano, parsley, and garlic powder.
3. Set your Instant Pot to Sauté and heat the coconut oil.
4. Sear each chicken breast until golden brown, about 4 to 5 minutes per side.
5. Remove the chicken breasts and set aside.
6. Pour the water into the Instant Pot and scrape the bottom to remove any chicken or seasoning that is stuck on. Add the trivet to the Instant Pot and place the chicken on the trivet.
7. Secure the lid. Select the Manual mode and set the cooking time for 15 minutes at High Pressure.
8. Once cooking is complete, do a natural pressure release for 15 minutes, then release any remaining pressure. Carefully open the lid. Serve warm.

Thai Peanut Chicken

Prep time: 6 mins, Cook time: 12 mins, Servings: 6

- 2 tbsps. chopped scallions
- Salt and pepper, to taste
- 1½ cups toasted peanuts, divided
- 2 garlic cloves, minced
- 1½ lbs. chicken breasts
- 1 cup water

1. Place 1 cup of toasted peanuts in a food processor and pulse until smooth. This will serve as your peanut butter.
2. On a flat work surface, chop the remaining toasted peanuts finely and set aside.
3. Press the Sauté button on the Instant Pot and add the chicken breasts and garlic. Keep on stirring for 3 minutes until the meat has turned lightly golden. Sprinkle pepper and salt for seasoning.
4. Pour in the prepared peanut butter and water. Give the mixture a good stir.
5. Lock the lid. Select the Poultry mode and set the cooking time for 8 minutes at High Pressure.
6. Once cooking is complete, do a natural pressure release for 5 minutes, then release any remaining pressure. Carefully open the lid.
7. Garnish with chopped peanuts and scallions before serving.

Thyme Chicken with Brussels Sprouts

Prep time: 10 mins, Cook Time: 25 mins, Servings: 4

- 1 tbsp. olive oil
- 2 chicken breasts, skinless, boneless and halved
- 2 cups Brussels sprouts, halved
- 1 cup chicken stock
- 2 thyme springs, chopped
- A pinch of salt and black pepper

1. Set your Instant Pot to Sauté and heat the olive oil. Add the chicken breasts and brown for 5 minutes.
2. Add the remaining ingredients to the pot and whisk to combine.
3. Lock the lid. Select the Poultry mode and set the cooking time for 20 minutes at High Pressure.
4. Once cooking is complete, do a natural pressure release for 10 minutes, then release any remaining pressure. Carefully open the lid.
5. Divide the chicken and Brussels sprouts among four plates and serve.

Whole Roasted Chicken with Lemon and Rosemary

Prep time: 2 hours, Cook time: 25 to 30 mins, Servings: 12

- 1 (5 to 6 pounds) whole chicken
- 6 minced garlic cloves
- Salt and pepper, to taste
- 1 sliced lemon
- 1 rosemary sprig
- 1 cup water or chicken broth

1. On a clean work surface, rub the chicken with the minced garlic cloves, salt and pepper.
2. Stuff the lemon slices and rosemary sprig into the cavity of the chicken. Place the chicken into the Instant Pot and add the water or chicken broth.
3. Lock the lid. Select the Poultry mode and cook for 25 to 30 minutes at High Pressure.
4. Once cooking is complete, do a natural pressure release for 15 minutes, then release any remaining pressure. Carefully open the lid.
5. Remove the chicken from the pot and shred it. Serve immediately.

CHAPTER 6 BEEF

Citrus Beef Carnitas

Prep time: 15 minutes | Cook time: 25 minutes | Serves 8

2½ pounds (1.1 kg) bone-in country ribs
Salt, to taste
¼ cup orange juice
1½ cups beef stock
1 onion, cut into wedges
2 garlic cloves, smashed and peeled
1 teaspoon chili powder
1 cup shredded Jack cheese

1. Season the ribs with salt on a clean work surface.
2. In the Instant Pot, combine the orange juice and stock. Fold in the onion and garlic. Put the ribs in the pot. Sprinkle with chili powder.
3. Seal the lid, select the Manual mode and set the cooking time for 25 minutes at High Pressure.
4. Once cooking is complete, do a natural pressure release for 10 minutes, then release any remaining pressure. Carefully open the lid. Transfer beef to a plate to cool.
5. Remove and discard the bones. Shred the ribs with two forks. Top the beef with the sauce remains in the pot. Sprinkled with cheese and serve.

Classic Pot Roast

Prep time: 15 minutes | Cook time: 1 hour 8 minutes | Serves 6

¼ cup dry red wine
1 tablespoon dried thyme
1½ cups beef broth
½ tablespoon dried rosemary
1 teaspoon paprika
1 teaspoon garlic powder
1½ teaspoons sea salt
½ teaspoon ground black pepper
3 pounds (1.4 kg) boneless chuck roast
1½ tablespoons avocado oil
2 tablespoons unsalted butter
½ medium yellow onion, chopped
2 garlic cloves, minced
1 cup sliced mushrooms
4 stalks celery, chopped
2 sprigs fresh thyme
1 bay leaf

1. In a medium bowl, combine the wine, dried thyme, beef broth, and dried rosemary. Stir to combine. Set aside.
2. In a small bowl, combine the paprika, garlic powder, sea salt, and black pepper. Mix well. Generously rub the dry spice mixture into the roast. Set aside.
3. Select Sauté mode. Once the pot becomes hot, add the avocado oil and butter and heat until the butter is melted, about 2 minutes.
4. Add the roast to the pot. Sauté for 3 minutes per side or until a crust is formed. Transfer the browned roast to a plate and set aside.
5. Add the onions and garlic to the pot. Sauté for 3 minutes or until the onions soften and the garlic becomes fragrant.
6. Add half the broth and wine mixture to the pot.
7. Place the trivet in the Instant Pot and place the roast on top of the trivet. Add the mushrooms and celery to the pot, and pour the remaining broth and wine mixture over the roast. Place the thyme sprigs and bay leaf on top of the roast.
8. Lock the lid. Select Manual mode and set cooking time for 1 hour on High Pressure.
9. When cooking is complete, allow the pressure to release naturally for 10 minutes and then release the remaining pressure.
10. Open the lid, discard the bay leaf and thyme sprigs. Transfer the roast to a serving platter.
11. Transfer the vegetables to the platter and spoon the remaining broth over the roast and vegetables.
12. Slice the roast and ladle ¼ cup of the broth over each serving. Serve hot.

Osso Buco with Gremolata

Prep time: 35 minutes | Cook time: 1 hour 2 minutes | Serves 6

4 bone-in beef shanks

Sea salt, to taste

2 tablespoons avocado oil

1 small turnip, diced

1 medium onion, diced

1 medium stalk celery, diced

4 cloves garlic, smashed

1 tablespoon unsweetened tomato purée

½ cup dry white wine

1 cup chicken broth

1 sprig fresh rosemary

2 sprigs fresh thyme

3 Roma tomatoes, diced

For the Gremolata:

½ cup loosely packed parsley leaves

1 clove garlic, crushed

Grated zest of 2 lemons

1. On a clean work surface, season the shanks all over with salt.

2. Set the Instant Pot to Sauté and add the oil. When the oil shimmers, add 2 shanks and sear for 4 minutes per side. Remove the shanks to a bowl and repeat with the remaining shanks. Set aside.

3. Add the turnip, onion, and celery to the pot and cook for 5 minutes or until softened.

4. Add the garlic and unsweetened tomato purée and cook 1 minute more, stirring frequently.

5. Deglaze the pot with the wine, scraping the bottom with a wooden spoon to loosen any browned bits. Bring to a boil.

6. Add the broth, rosemary, thyme, and shanks, then add the tomatoes on top of the shanks.

7. Secure the lid. Press the Manual button and set cooking time for 40 minutes on High Pressure.

8. Meanwhile, for the gremolata: In a small food processor, combine the parsley, garlic, and lemon zest and pulse until the parsley is finely chopped. Refrigerate until ready to use.

9. When timer beeps, allow the pressure to release naturally for 20 minutes, then release any remaining pressure. Open the lid.

10. To serve, transfer the shanks to large, shallow serving bowl. Ladle the braising sauce over the top and sprinkle with the gremolata.

Sloppy Joes

Prep time: 10 minutes | Cook time: 19 minutes | Serves 4

1 pound (454 g) ground beef, divided

½ cup chopped onion

½ cup chopped green bell pepper

¼ cup water

2 teaspoons Worcestershire sauce

1 garlic clove, minced

1 tablespoon Dijon mustard

¾ cup ketchup

2 teaspoons brown sugar

¼ teaspoon sea salt

½ teaspoon hot sauce

4 soft hamburger buns

1. Select the Sauté mode of the Instant Pot. Put about ½ cup of the ground beef in the pot and cook for about 4 minutes or until browned.

2. Stir in the onion, bell pepper, and water. Add the remaining beef and cook for about 3 minutes or until well browned.

3. Mix in the Worcestershire sauce, garlic, mustard, ketchup, brown sugar, and salt.

4. Lock the lid. Select the Manual mode. Set the time for 12 minutes at High Pressure.

5. When timer beeps, quick release the pressure, then unlock the lid.

6. Stir in the hot sauce. Select the Sauté mode and simmer until lightly thickened. Spoon the meat and sauce into the buns. Serve immediately.

Corned Beef

Prep time: 6 mins, Cook Time: 1 hour 30 mins, Servings: 4

- 12 oz. beer
- 1 cup water
- 3 garlic cloves, minced
- 3 lbs. corned beef brisket
- Salt and pepper, to taste

1. Pour the beer and water into the Instant Pot. Add the garlic and mix to combine well.
2. Put the steamer basket inside.
3. Add the beef to the basket and season with salt and pepper.
4. Cover the pot. Select the Meat/Stew mode and cook at High Pressure for 90 minutes.
5. Once cooking is complete, do a quick pressure release for 10 minutes, and then release any remaining pressure. Carefully open the lid.
6. Transfer the beef to a baking pan and cover it with foil.
7. Let it rest for 15 minutes before slicing to serve.

Japanese Beef Shanks

Prep time: 15 minutes | Cook time: 30 minutes | Serves 4

1 pound (454 g) beef shank

½ teaspoon Five-spice powder

1 teaspoon instant dashi granules

½ teaspoon garlic, minced

1 tablespoon tamari or soy sauce

¼ cup rice wine

1 clove star anise

½ dried red chili, sliced

1 tablespoon sesame oil

¾ cup water

1. Combine all ingredients to the Instant Pot.
2. Secure the lid. Choose the Manual mode and set the cooking time for 30 minutes at High pressure.
3. Once cooking is complete, use a natural pressure release for 10 minutes, then release any remaining pressure. Carefully open the lid.

4. Slice the beef shank and serve hot.

Garlicky Prime Rib

Prep time: 12 mins, Cook Time: 1 hour, Servings: 10

- 2 tbsps. olive oil
- 10 garlic cloves, minced
- 4 lbs. prime rib roast
- 2 tsps. dried thyme
- Salt and pepper, to taste
- 1 cup water

1. Press the Sauté button on the Instant Pot and heat the oil.
2. Add and sauté the garlic for 1 to 2 minutes until fragrant.
3. Add the prime rib roast and sear on all sides for 3 minutes until lightly browned.
4. Sprinkle with thyme, salt and pepper.
5. Pour in the water and remove the browning at the bottom.
6. Lock the lid. Set the pot to Meat/Stew mode and set the timer to 1 hour at High Pressure.
7. Once cooking is complete, use a natural pressure release for 10 minutes, then release any remaining pressure.
8. Carefully open the lid. Allow to cool for a few minutes. Transfer them on a large plate and serve immediately.

Beef with Garlic

Prep time: 12 mins, Cook time: 10 mins, Servings: 4

- 1½ lbs. beef sirloin
- 1 tbsp. sea salt
- 1 tbsp. extra virgin olive oil
- 5 garlic cloves, chopped
- 1 cup heavy cream

1. On a clean work surface, rub the beef with salt.
2. Set the Instant Pot to Sauté mode. Add the olive oil and heat until shimmering.
3. Add the beef and sear for 3 minutes until lightly browned.
4. Add garlic and sauté for 30 seconds or until fragrant.
5. Mix in the heavy cream.

6. Lock the lid. Set the pot to Manual setting and set the timer for 10 minutes at High Pressure.

7. When the timer beeps, press Cancel, then use a natural pressure release for 10 minutes, and then release any remaining pressure.

8. Carefully open the lid. Allow to cool for a few minutes. Transfer them on a large plate and serve immediately.

Ginger Short Ribs

Prep time: 12 mins, Cook Time: 25 mins, Servings: 6

- 4 beef short ribs
- 1 tsp. salt
- 3 tbsps. extra virgin olive oil, plus 1 tbsp. for coating
- 1 large onion, diced
- 2-inch knob of ginger, grated
- ¾ cup water

1. On a clean work surface, rub the ribs with salt.

2. Lightly coat the Instant Pot with olive oil and set the setting to Sauté.

3. Add the onion and ginger, then sauté for a minute

4. Add the ribs and brown for 4 to 5 minutes. Pour in the water.

5. Lock the lid. Set to Manual mode and set the cooking time for 25 minutes at High Pressure.

6. Once cooking is complete, use a natural pressure release for 10 minutes, then release any remaining pressure.

7. Carefully open the lid. Allow to cool for a few minutes. Transfer them on a large plate and serve immediately.

Gingered Beef Tenderloin

Prep time: 12 mins, Cook Time: 1 hour, Servings: 8

- 2 tbsps. olive oil
- 2 tbsps. minced garlic
- 2 tbsps. thinly sliced ginger
- 4 fillet mignon steaks
- ¼ cup soy sauce
- Salt and pepper, to taste
- 1 cup water

1. Press the Sauté button on the Instant Pot and heat the olive oil.

2. Sauté the garlic for 1 minute until fragrant.

3. Add the ginger and fillet mignon and allow to sear for 4 minutes or until lightly browned.

4. Drizzle with the soy sauce. Add salt and pepper to taste. Pour in a cup of water.

5. Lock the lid and select the Meat/Stew mode and set the timer to 1 hour at High Pressure.

6. Once cooking is complete, use a natural pressure release for 10 minutes, then release any remaining pressure.

7. Carefully open the lid. Allow to cool for a few minutes. Transfer them on a large plate and discard the bay leaf, then serve.

Greek Beef and Spinach Ravioli

Prep time: 15 minutes | Cook time: 20 minutes | Serves 4

1 cup cheese ravioli

3 cups water

Salt, to taste

1 tablespoon olive oil

1 pound (454 g) ground beef

1 cup canned diced tomatoes

1 tablespoon dried mixed herbs

3 cups chicken broth

1 cup baby spinach

¼ cup Kalamata olives, sliced

¼ cup crumbled feta cheese

1. Put ravioli, water, and salt in Instant Pot. Seal the lid, select the Manual mode and set the time for 3 minutes at High Pressure.

2. Once cooking is complete, do a quick pressure release. Carefully open the lid. Drain the ravioli through a colander and set aside.

3. Set the pot to Sauté mode, then heat the olive oil. Add and brown the beef for 5 minutes.

4. Mix in the tomatoes, mixed herbs, and chicken broth. Seal the lid, select the Manual mode and set cooking time for 10 minutes on High Pressure.

5. When timer beeps, do a quick pressure release. Carefully open the lid.

6. Set the pot to Sauté mode, then mix in ravioli, spinach, olives and cook for 2 minutes or until spinach wilts. Stir in the feta cheese and serve.

Mushroom Beef Stroganoff

Prep time: 25 minutes | Cook time: 20 minutes | Serves 8

2 pounds (907 g) ground beef, divided

1½ teaspoons salt, divided

1 teaspoon ground black pepper, divided

½ pound (227 g) sliced fresh mushrooms

1 tablespoon butter

2 medium onions, chopped

2 garlic cloves, minced

1 (10½-ounce / 298-g) can condensed beef consomme, undiluted

⅓ cup all-purpose flour

2 tablespoons tomato paste

1½ cups sour cream

Hot cooked noodles, for serving

1. Select the Sauté setting of the Instant Pot. Add half of ground beef, salt and pepper. Sauté for 8 minutes or until no longer pink. Remove the beef. Repeat with remaining ground beef, salt and pepper.
2. Add mushrooms, butter, and onions to Instant Pot. Sauté for 6 minutes or until mushrooms are tender. Add garlic and sauté for 1 minute more until fragrant. Return the beef to the pot.
3. Lock the lid. Select the Manual setting and set the cooking time for 5 minutes at High Pressure.
4. When timer beeps, quick release pressure. Carefully open the lid. Select the Sauté setting.
5. In a small bowl, whisk together consomme, flour and tomato paste. Pour over the beef and stir to combine.
6. Sauté for 3 more minutes or until thickened. Stir in sour cream; cook for a minute more until heated through. Serve with noodles.

Beef Ribs with Leek

Prep time: 40 minutes | Cook time: 1 hour 40 minutes | Serves 4

1 pound (454 g) beef short ribs, bone-in

½ medium leek, sliced

½ teaspoon celery seeds

1 teaspoon onion soup mix

1 clove garlic, sliced

1 sprig thyme

1 sprig rosemary

1 tablespoon olive oil

Sea salt and ground black pepper, to taste

1 cup water

1. Place all ingredients in the Instant Pot.
2. Secure the lid. Choose the Manual mode and set the cooking time for 90 minutes at High pressure.
3. Once cooking is complete, do a natural pressure release for 30 minutes, then release any remaining pressure. Carefully open the lid.
4. Transfer the short ribs in the broiler and broil for 10 minutes or until crispy.
5. Transfer the ribs to a platter and serve.

Herbed Sirloin Tip Roast

Prep time: 5 mins, Cook Time: 1 hour 30 mins, Servings: 6

- 2 tbsps. mixed herbs
- 1 tsp. garlic powder
- 3 lbs. sirloin tip roast
- 1¼ tsps. paprika
- 1 cup water
- Salt and pepper, to taste

1. In the Instant Pot, combine all the ingredients. Stir to mix well.
2. Lock the lid. Set the pot to Meat/Stew mode and set the timer to 1 hour 30 minutes at High Pressure.
3. Once cooking is complete, use a natural pressure release for 10 minutes, then release any remaining pressure.
4. Carefully open the lid. Allow to cool for a few minutes. Transfer them on a large plate and discard the bay leaf, then serve.

Sirloin with Snap Peas

Prep time: 15 minutes | Cook time: 8 minutes | Serves 4

½ teaspoon hot sauce

1 teaspoon balsamic vinegar

1 cup chicken stock

¼ cup soy sauce

2 tablespoons sesame oil, divided

2 tablespoons maple syrup

½ cup plus 2 teaspoons cornstarch, divided

1 pound (454 g) beef sirloin, sliced

2 cups snap peas

3 garlic cloves, minced

3 scallions, sliced

1. In a bowl, combine the hot sauce, vinegar, stock, soy sauce, 1 tablespoon of sesame oil, maple syrup, and 2 tablespoons of cornstarch. Set aside.

2. Pour the remaining cornstarch on a plate. Season beef with salt, and pepper; toss lightly in cornstarch.

3. Set the Instant Pot to Sauté mode, heat the remaining sesame oil and fry the beef in batches for 5 minutes or until browned and crispy. Remove the beef from the pot and set aside.

4. Wipe the Instant Pot clean and pour in hot sauce mixture. Return meat to the pot, then add snow peas and garlic.

5. Seal the lid, select the Manual mode and set the time for 3 minutes on High Pressure.

6. When cooking is complete, perform natural pressure release for 10 minutes, then release the remaining pressure. Unlock the lid.

7. Dish out and garnish with scallions.

Indian Spicy Beef with Basmati

Prep time: 15 minutes | Cook time: 15 minutes | Serves 4

1 tablespoon olive oil

1 pound (454 g) beef stew meat, cubed

Salt and black pepper, to taste

½ teaspoon garam masala powder

½ teaspoon grated ginger

2 white onions, sliced

2 garlic cloves, minced

1 tablespoon cilantro leaves

½ teaspoon red chili powder

1 teaspoon cumin powder

¼ teaspoon turmeric powder

1 cup basmati rice

1 cup grated carrots

2 cups beef broth

¼ cup cashew nuts

¼ cup coconut yogurt, for serving

1. Set the Instant Pot to Sauté mode, then heat the olive oil.

2. Season the beef with salt and pepper, and brown both sides for 5 minutes. Transfer to a plate and set aside.

3. Add and sauté the garam masala, ginger, onions, garlic, cilantro, red chili, cumin, turmeric, salt, and pepper for 2 minutes.

4. Stir in beef, rice, carrots, and broth. Seal the lid, select the Manual mode, and set the time to 6 minutes on High Pressure.

5. When cooking is complete, do a natural pressure release for 5 minutes, then release any remaining pressure. Unlock the lid.

6. Fluff the rice and stir in cashews. Serve with coconut yogurt.

Instant Pot Rib Roast

Prep time: 6 mins, Cook Time: 2 hours 30 mins, Servings: 12

- 5 lbs. beef rib roast
- 1 tsp. garlic powder
- 1 bay leaf
- 1 tbsp. olive oil
- Salt and pepper, to taste
- 1 cup water

1. Put all the ingredients in the Instant Pot. Stir to mix well.

2. Lock the lid. Set the pot to Meat/Stew mode and set the timer to 2 hours 30 minutes at High Pressure.

3. Once cooking is complete, use a natural pressure release for 10 to 20 minutes, then release any remaining pressure.

4. Carefully open the lid. Allow to cool for a few minutes. Transfer them on a large plate and discard the bay leaf, then serve.

Korean Beef Ribs

Prep time: 10 minutes | Cook time: 15 minutes | Serves 6

3 pounds (1.4 kg) beef short ribs
1 cup beef broth
2 green onions, sliced
1 tablespoon toasted sesame seeds
Sauce:
½ teaspoon gochujang
½ cup rice wine
½ cup soy sauce
½ teaspoon garlic powder
½ teaspoon ground ginger
½ cup pure maple syrup
1 teaspoon white pepper
1 tablespoon sesame oil

1. In a large bowl, combine the ingredients for the sauce. Dunk the rib in the bowl and press to coat well. Cover the bowl in plastic and refrigerate for at least an hour.
2. Add the beef broth to the Instant Pot. Insert a trivet. Arrange the ribs standing upright over the trivet. Lock the lid.
3. Press the Manual button and set the cooking time for 25 minutes at High Pressure.
4. When timer beeps, let pressure release naturally for 10 minutes, then release any remaining pressure. Unlock the lid.
5. Transfer ribs to a serving platter and garnish with green onions and sesame seeds. Serve immediately.

Lemon Beef Meal

Prep time: 12 mins, Cook Time: 10 mins, Servings: 2
- 1 tbsp. olive oil
- 2 beef steaks
- ½ tsp. garlic salt
- 1 garlic clove, crushed
- 2 tbsps. lemon juice

1. Press Sauté on the Instant Pot. Heat the olive oil in the pot until shimmering.
2. Add the beef and garlic salt and sauté for 4 to 5 minutes to evenly brown.

3. Add the garlic and sauté for 1 minute until fragrant.
4. Serve with lemon juice on top.

Lemongrass Rice and Beef Pot

Prep time: 45 minutes | Cook time: 15 minutes | Serves 4

1 pound (454 g) beef stew meat, cut into cubes
2 tablespoons olive oil
1 green bell pepper, chopped
1 red bell pepper, chopped
1 lemongrass stalk, sliced
1 onion, chopped
2 garlic cloves, minced
1 cup jasmine rice
2 cups chicken broth
2 tablespoons chopped parsley, for garnish
Marinade:
1 tablespoon rice wine
½ teaspoon Five-spice
½ teaspoon miso paste
1 teaspoon garlic purée
1 teaspoon chili powder
1 teaspoon cumin powder
1 tablespoon soy sauce
1 teaspoon plus ½ tablespoon ginger paste, divided
½ teaspoon sesame oil
Salt and black pepper, to taste

1. In a bowl, add beef and top with the ingredients for the marinade. Mix and wrap the bowl in plastic. Marinate in the refrigerator for 30 minutes.
2. Set the Instant Pot to Sauté mode, then heat the olive oil.
3. Drain beef from marinade and brown in the pot for 5 minutes. Flip frequently.
4. Stir in bell peppers, lemongrass, onion, and garlic. Sauté for 3 minutes.
5. Stir in rice, cook for 1 minute. Pour in the broth. Seal the lid, select the Manual mode and set the time for 5 minutes on High Pressure.
6. When timer beeps, perform a quick pressure release. Carefully open the lid.
7. Dish out and garnish with parsley. Serve warm.

Mexican Beef Shred

Prep time: 20 minutes | Cook time: 30 minutes | Serves 4

1 pound (454 g) tender chuck roast, cut into half
3 tablespoons chipotle sauce
1 (8-ounce / 227-g) can tomato sauce
1 cup beef broth
½ cup chopped cilantro
1 lime, zested and juiced
2 teaspoons cumin powder
1 teaspoon cayenne pepper
Salt and ground black pepper, to taste
½ teaspoon garlic powder
1 tablespoon olive oil

1. In the Instant Pot, add the beef, chipotle sauce, tomato sauce, beef broth, cilantro, lime zest, lime juice, cumin powder, cayenne pepper, salt, pepper, and garlic powder.
2. Seal the lid, then select the Manual mode and set the cooking time for 30 minutes at High Pressure.
3. Once cooking is complete, allow a natural pressure release for 10 minutes, then release any remaining pressure.
4. Unlock the lid and using two forks to shred the beef into strands. Stir in the olive oil. Serve warm.

Sautéed Beef and Green Beans

Prep time: 12 mins, Cook Time: 5 mins, Servings: 4

*   1 tbsp. olive oil
*   10 oz. fat removed beef sirloin
*   2 spring onions, chopped
*   7 oz. canned green beans
*   2 tbsps. soy sauce
*   Salt and pepper, to taste

1. Press Sauté on the Instant Pot. Grease the pot with the olive oil.
2. Add the beef and sauté for 2 to 3 minutes to evenly brown.
3. Add the onions, green beans, and soy sauce, then sauté for another 2 to 3 minutes until the beans are soft. Sprinkle with salt and pepper.

4. Serve warm.

Herbed Beef Chuck Roast

Prep time: 15 minutes | Cook time: 1 hour | Serves 8

2 tablespoons coconut oil
3 pounds (1.4 kg) beef chuck roast
1 cup water
½ teaspoon dried parsley
½ teaspoon dried basil
½ teaspoon chili powder
½ teaspoon fresh paprika
1 cup butter
½ teaspoon kosher salt
½ teaspoon freshly ground black pepper

1. Set the Instant Pot to Sauté mode and melt the coconut oil.
2. Add and sear the roast for 4 minutes or until browned on both sides. Flip the roast halfway through, then remove from the pot.
3. Pour the water into the Instant Pot, then add the parsley, basil, chili powder, paprika, butter, salt, and black pepper. Return the beef to the pot.
4. Close the lid. Select the Manual mode, set the cooking time for 55 minutes on High Pressure.
5. When timer beeps, naturally release the pressure for about 10 minutes, then release any remaining pressure. Open the lid.
6. Serve immediately.

Slow Cooked Beef Pizza Casserole

Prep time: 15 minutes | Cook time: 3 hours 4 minutes | Serves 6

2 tablespoons olive oil, divided
1 pound (454 g) ground beef
2 cups shredded whole Mozzarella cheese, divided
1 tablespoon Italian seasoning blend, divided
1 teaspoon garlic powder, divided
½ cup unsweetened tomato purée
¼ teaspoon dried oregano
¼ teaspoon sea salt
15 slices pepperoni
2 tablespoons sliced black olives

1. Select Sauté mode. Once the pot is hot, add 1 tablespoon olive oil and crumble the ground beef into the pot. Sauté for 4 minutes until the meat is browned.
2. Place a colander over a large bowl. Transfer the meat to the colander to drain and then transfer the drained meat to a large mixing bowl.
3. To the bowl with the meat, add 1 cup Mozzarella, ½ tablespoon Italian seasoning, and ½ teaspoon garlic powder. Mix until well combined. Set aside.
4. In a small bowl, combine the tomato purée, remaining Italian seasoning, remaining garlic powder, oregano, and sea salt. Mix well. Set aside.
5. Coat the bottom of the Instant Pot with the remaining olive oil. Press the meat mixture into the bottom of the pot.
6. Add the tomato purée mixture to the pot and use a spoon to evenly distribute the sauce over the meat. Add the pepperoni over the sauce. Sprinkle the remaining Mozzarella over and then top with the olives.
7. Lock the lid. Select Slow Cook mode and set cooking time for 3 hours on Normal.
8. When cooking is complete, open the lid and transfer the casserole to a serving platter. Slice into six equal-sized wedges. Serve hot.

Slow Cooked Beef Steak

Prep time: 10 minutes | Cook time: 7 hours | Serves 4
½ cup butter, softened
1 pound (454 g) beef steak
1 teaspoon ground nutmeg
½ teaspoon salt
1. Heat the butter in the Instant Pot on Sauté mode.
2. When the butter is melted, add beef steak, ground nutmeg, and salt.
3. Close the lid and select Slow Cook mode and set cooking time for 7 hours on Less.
4. When cooking is complete, allow to cool for half an hour and serve warm.

Steak and Bell Pepper Fajitas

Prep time: 15 minutes | Cook time: 45 minutes | Serves 6

1 (2-pound / 907-g) skirt steak
1 medium red bell pepper, deseeded and diced
1 medium green bell pepper, deseeded and diced
1 small onion, diced
1 cup beef broth
Sauce:
1 tablespoon fish sauce
¼ cup soy sauce
1 teaspoon ground cumin
2 tablespoons tomato paste
1 teaspoon chili powder
½ teaspoon sea salt
⅛ cup avocado oil
1. In a small bowl, combine the ingredients for the sauce. Spread ¾ of the sauce on all sides of the beef on a clean work surface. Reserve the remaining sauce.
2. Press the Sauté button on Instant Pot. Add skirt steak and sear on each side for about 5 minutes. Remove the meat and set aside.
3. Add the bell peppers and onion with reserved sauce. Sauté for 3 to 5 minutes or until the onions are translucent.
4. Pour in the beef broth. Set the beef over the onion and peppers. Lock the lid.
5. Press the Meat / Stew button and set the cooking time for 35 minutes at High Pressure.
6. When timer beeps, let the pressure release naturally for 15 minutes, then release any remaining pressure. Unlock the lid.
7. Using a slotted spoon, remove the meat and vegetables to a serving platter. Thinly slice the skirt steak and serve.

Steak, Pepper, and Lettuce Salad

Prep time: 20 minutes | Cook time: 25 minutes | Serves 4
¾ pound (340 g) steak
¼ cup red wine
½ teaspoon red pepper flakes
Sea salt and ground black pepper, to taste
¾ cup water
2 tablespoons olive oil
1 tablespoon wine vinegar

1 sweet pepper, cut into strips

½ red onion, sliced

1 butterhead lettuce, separate into leaves

¼ cup feta cheese, crumbled

¼ cup black olives, pitted and sliced

1. Add the steak, red wine, red pepper, salt, black pepper, and water to the Instant Pot.

2. Secure the lid. Choose the Manual mode and set the cooking time for 25 minutes at High pressure.

3. Once cooking is complete, perform a natural pressure release for 10 minutes. Carefully open the lid.

4. Thinly slice the steak and transfer to a salad bowl. Toss with the olive oil and vinegar.

5. Add the peppers, red onion, and lettuce, then toss to combine well. Top with cheese and olives and serve.

Sumptuous Beef and Tomato Biryani

Prep time: 10 minutes | Cook time: 25 minutes | Serves 6

1 tablespoon ghee

1 small onion, sliced

1 pound (454 g) top round, cut into strips

1 (28-ounce / 794-g) can whole stewed tomatoes, with juice

1 cup plain Greek yogurt

1 tablespoon minced fresh ginger root

2 cloves garlic, minced

½ teaspoon ground cloves

½ teaspoon ground cumin

½ teaspoon ground coriander

½ teaspoon ground cinnamon

½ teaspoon ground cardamom

1 teaspoon salt

½ teaspoon ground black pepper

2 cups cooked basmati rice

1. Press the Sauté button on Instant Pot. Melt the ghee.

2. Add the onion and sauté for 3 to 5 minutes or until translucent.

3. Add the remaining ingredients, except for the rice, to the Instant Pot. Lock the lid.

4. Press the Manual button and set the cooking time for 10 minutes at High Pressure.

5. When timer beeps, quick release the pressure, then unlock the lid.

6. Press the Sauté button and simmer for about 10 minutes or until most of the liquid has evaporated. Serve over cooked basmati rice.

Super Beef Chili

Prep time: 12 mins, Cook Time: 8 mins, Servings: 4

- 1 lb. ground beef
- 1½ tsps. sea salt
- 1 medium onion, chopped
- 2 cups tomato purée
- 2 cups zucchini, peeled and rinsed, cut into 1-inch bites
- 1 cup water
- 1 tsp. chili spice powder

1. Select the Instant Pot to Sauté setting. Coat the pot with olive oil and heat until shimmering.

2. Add the beef, salt and onion, then sauté for 4 minutes or until the beef is lightly browned.

3. Add the tomato purée, zucchini, water and chili spice powder. Stir to mix well.

4. Lock the lid. Set the Instant Pot to Manual setting and set the timer for 8 minutes at High Pressure.

5. Once cooking is complete, use a quick pressure release.

6. Carefully open the lid. Allow to cool for a few minutes. Transfer them on a large plate and serve immediately.

Sweet Apricot Beef

Prep time: 12 mins, Cook Time: 30 mins, Servings: 4

- 1½ lbs. beef tenderloin
- 1 tsp. sea salt
- 1 tbsp. coconut oil
- 4 apricots, pitted and sliced thinly
- ½ cup chopped almonds
- 1 cup water

1. On a clean work surface, sprinkle the beef with salt and cut into 1-inch thick slices.

2. Set the Instant Pot to Sauté setting, then add coconut oil and heat until melted.

3. Add the beef and sauté for 4 to 5 minutes or until browned.

4. Add the apricot and sauté for a minute. Add the chopped almonds. Pour in the water.

5. Lock the lid. Press the Manual setting and set the timer at 30 minutes at High Pressure.

6. When the timer beeps, press Cancel, then use a quick pressure release.

7. Carefully open the lid and allow to cool for a few minutes. Serve warm.

Sweet Potato Beef

Prep time: 12 mins, Cook Time: 40 mins, Servings: 4

- 1 tbsp. olive oil
- 1 lb. lean beef stew meat
- 4 cups low-sodium beef stock
- 1 small sweet potato, diced
- 1 tomato, roughly chopped
- 2 bell peppers, sliced
- Salt and pepper, to taste

1. Press Sauté on Instant Pot. Grease the pot with the olive oil.

2. Add the beef and sauté for 4 to 5 minutes to evenly brown.

3. Mix in the remaining ingredients.

4. Lock the lid. Press Manual. Set the timer to 35 minutes at High Pressure.

5. When the timer beeps, press Cancel, then use a quick pressure release.

6. Open the lid, transfer them in 4 plates and serve warm.

Tequila Short Ribs

Prep time: 3 hours 25 minutes | Cook time: 35 minutes | Serves 4

1 pound (454 g) chuck short ribs
1 shot tequila
½ tablespoon stone ground mustard
½ tablespoon Sriracha sauce
½ cup apple cider
1 tablespoon tomato paste
1 tablespoon honey

½ teaspoon marjoram
½ teaspoon garlic powder
½ teaspoon shallot powder
½ teaspoon paprika
Kosher salt and cracked black pepper, to taste
¾ cup beef bone broth

1. Place all ingredients, except for the beef broth, in a large bowl. Cover with a foil and let it marinate for 3 hours in the refrigerator.

2. Pour the beef along with the marinade in the Instant Pot. Pour in the beef bone broth.

3. Secure the lid. Choose the Meat / Stew mode and set the cooking time for 35 minutes at High pressure.

4. Once cooking is complete, do a natural pressure release for 15 minutes, then release any remaining pressure. Carefully open the lid.

5. Serve immediately.

Thai Coconut Beef with Snap Peas

Prep time: 30 minutes | Cook time: 40 minutes | Serves 10

1 (3-pound / 1.4-kg) boneless beef chuck roast, halved
1 teaspoon salt
1 teaspoon ground black pepper
2 tablespoons canola oil
1 (14-ounce / 397-g) can coconut milk
½ cup creamy peanut butter
¼ cup red curry paste
2 tablespoons honey
¾ cup beef stock
2 tablespoons soy sauce
2 teaspoons minced fresh ginger root
1 large sweet red pepper, sliced
½ pound (227 g) fresh sugar snap peas, trimmed
¼ cup minced fresh cilantro

1. Sprinkle the beef with salt and pepper on a clean work surface. Select the Sauté setting of the Instant Pot. Add the canola oil and heat.

2. Add one roast half. Brown on all sides for about 5 minutes. Remove and repeat with remaining beef half.

3. Meanwhile, in a bowl, whisk the coconut milk with peanut butter, curry paste, honey, beef stock, soy sauce, and ginger root.

4. Put all the beef halves into the Instant Pot, then add red pepper and pour the coconut milk mixture over the beef.

5. Lock the lid. Select the Manual setting and set the cooking time for 35 minutes at High Pressure.

6. When timer beeps, quick release the pressure. Carefully open the lid.

7. Add the sugar snap peas and set the cooking time for 5 minutes at High Pressure.

8. When timer beeps, naturally release the pressure for 10 minutes, then release any remaining pressure. Unlock the lid.

9. Remove beef from the pot. Skim fat from cooking juices. Shred beef with forks. Stir in cilantro and serve.

Winter Beef Roast Pot

Prep time: 15 minutes | Cook time: 40 minutes | Serves 6

2 tablespoons olive oil
1 (3-pound / 1.4-kg) chuck roast
½ cup dry red wine
1 (1-pound / 454-g) butternut squash, chopped
2 carrots, chopped
¾ cup pearl onions
1 teaspoon dried oregano leaves
1 bay leaf
1½ cups beef broth
Salt and black pepper, to taste
1 small red onion, quartered

1. Select the Sauté mode of the Instant Pot and heat the olive oil.

2. Season the beef with salt and sear in the pot for 3 minutes per side or until well browned.

3. Mix in the wine. Bring to a boil and cook for 2 more minutes or until the wine has reduced by half.

4. Mix in the butternut squash, carrots, pearl onions, oregano, bay leaf, broth, black pepper, and red onion. Stir to combine and add the beef.

5. Seal the lid, then select the Manual mode and set the time for 35 minutes on High Pressure.

6. Once cooking is complete, do a quick pressure release. Carefully open the lid.

7. Remove the beef and slice. Spoon over the sauce and vegetables to serve.

CHAPTER 7 PORK

Pork Steaks with Pico de Gallo

Prep time: 15 minutes | Cook time: 12 minutes | Serves 6

1 tablespoon butter
2 pounds (907 g) pork steaks
1 bell pepper, deseeded and sliced
½ cup shallots, chopped
2 garlic cloves, minced
¼ cup dry red wine
1 cup chicken bone broth
¼ cup water
Salt, to taste
¼ teaspoon freshly ground black pepper, or more to taste
Pico de Gallo:
1 tomato, chopped
1 chili pepper, seeded and minced
½ cup red onion, chopped
2 garlic cloves, minced
1 tablespoon fresh cilantro, finely chopped
Sea salt, to taste

1. Press the Sauté button to heat up the Instant Pot. Melt the butter and sear the pork steaks about 4 minutes or until browned on both sides.
2. Add bell pepper, shallot, garlic, wine, chicken bone broth, water, salt, and black pepper to the Instant Pot.
3. Secure the lid. Choose the Manual mode and set cooking time for 8 minutes at High pressure.
4. Meanwhile, combine the ingredients for the Pico de Gallo in a small bowl. Refrigerate until ready to serve.
5. Once cooking is complete, use a quick pressure release. Carefully remove the lid.
6. Serve warm pork steaks with the chilled Pico de Gallo on the side.

Egg Meatloaf

Prep time: 20 minutes | Cook time: 25 minutes | Serves 6

1 tablespoon avocado oil
1½ cup ground pork
1 teaspoon chives
1 teaspoon salt
½ teaspoon ground black pepper
2 tablespoons coconut flour
3 eggs, hard-boiled, peeled
1 cup water

1. Brush a loaf pan with avocado oil.
2. In the mixing bowl, mix the ground pork, chives, salt, ground black pepper, and coconut flour.
3. Transfer the mixture in the loaf pan and flatten with a spatula.
4. Fill the meatloaf with hard-boiled eggs.
5. Pour water and insert the trivet in the Instant Pot.
6. Lower the loaf pan over the trivet in the Instant Pot. Close the lid.
7. Select Manual mode and set cooking time for 25 minutes on High Pressure.
8. When timer beeps, use a natural pressure release for 10 minutes, then release any remaining pressure. Open the lid.
9. Serve immediately.

Eggplant Pork Lasagna

Prep time: 20 minutes | Cook time: 30 minutes | Serves 6

2 eggplants, sliced
1 teaspoon salt
10 ounces (283 g) ground pork
1 cup Mozzarella, shredded
1 tablespoon unsweetened tomato purée
1 teaspoon butter, softened
1 cup chicken stock

1. Sprinkle the eggplants with salt and let sit for 10 minutes, then pat dry with paper towels.
2. In a mixing bowl, mix the ground pork, butter, and tomato purée.
3. Make a layer of the sliced eggplants in the bottom of the Instant Pot and top with ground pork mixture.
4. Top the ground pork with Mozzarella and repeat with remaining ingredients.

5. Pour in the chicken stock. Close the lid. Select Manual mode and set cooking time for 30 minutes on High Pressure.
6. When timer beeps, use a natural pressure release for 10 minutes, then release the remaining pressure and open the lid.
7. Cool for 10 minutes and serve.

Garlicky Pork Tenderloin

Prep time: 6 mins, Cook Time: 8 hours, Servings: 10
- 3 tbsps. extra virgin olive oil
- ¼ cup butter
- 1 tsp. thyme
- 1 garlic clove, minced
- 3 lbs. pork tenderloin
- 1 cup water
- Salt and pepper, to taste

1. Set the Instant Pot on Sauté. Heat the olive oil and butter until the butter is melted.
2. Add and sauté the garlic and thyme for 1 minute or until fragrant.
3. Add the pork tenderloin and sauté for 3 minutes or until lightly browned.
4. Pour in the water and sprinkle salt and pepper for seasoning.
5. Lock the lid. Press the Slow Cook button and set the cooking time to 8 hours at High Pressure.
6. Once cooking is complete, perform a natural pressure release for 10 minutes, and then release any remaining pressure. Carefully open the lid.
7. Allow to cool for a few minutes. Remove the pork from the pot and serve warm.

Golden Bacon Sticks

Prep time: 5 minutes | Cook time: 6 minutes | Serves 4
6 ounces (170 g) bacon, sliced
2 tablespoons almond flour
1 tablespoon water
¾ teaspoon chili pepper
1. Sprinkle the sliced bacon with the almond flour and drizzle with water. Add the chili pepper.
2. Put the bacon in the Instant Pot.

3. Cook on Sauté mode for 3 minutes per side.
4. Serve immediately.

Hawaiian Pulled Pork Roast with Cabbage

Prep time: 10 minutes | Cook time: 1 hour 2 minutes minutes | Serves 6
1½ tablespoons olive oil
3 pounds (1.4 kg) pork shoulder roast, cut into 4 equal-sized pieces
3 cloves garlic, minced
1 tablespoon liquid smoke
2 cups water, divided
1 tablespoon sea salt
2 cups shredded cabbage
1. Select Sauté mode and add the olive oil to the Instant Pot. Once the oil is hot, add the pork cuts and sear for 5 minutes per side or until browned. Once browned, transfer the pork to a platter and set aside.
2. Add the garlic, liquid smoke, and 1½ cups water to the Instant Pot. Stir to combine.
3. Return the pork to the pot and sprinkle the salt over top.
4. Lock the lid. Select Manual mode and set cooking time for 1 hour on High Pressure.
5. When cooking is complete, allow the pressure to release naturally for 20 minutes, then release any remaining pressure.
6. Open the lid and transfer the pork to a large platter. Using two forks, shred the pork. Set aside.
7. Add the shredded cabbage and remaining water to the liquid in the pot. Stir.
8. Lock the lid. Select Manual mode and set cooking time for 2 minutes on High Pressure. When cooking is complete, quick release the pressure.
9. Transfer the cabbage to the serving platter with the pork. Serve warm.

Barbecue-Honey Baby Back Ribs

Prep time: 10 minutes | Cook time: 25 minutes | Serves 4

2 racks baby back ribs (3 pounds / 1.4 kg; about 4 ribs each), cut into 5- to 6-inch portions
2 tablespoons chili powder
2 tablespoons toasted sesame oil
3 tablespoons grainy mustard
1 tablespoon red wine vinegar
1 cup ketchup
⅓ cup honey
½ cup chicken broth

1. Rub the ribs all over with the chili powder.
2. Mix together the remaining ingredients in your Instant Pot and stir until the honey has dissolved.
3. Dip the ribs in the sauce to coat. Using tongs, arrange the ribs standing upright against the sides of the pot.
4. Secure the lid. Select the Manual function and cook for 25 minutes on High Pressure.
5. Preheat the broiler and adjust an oven rack so that it is 4 inches below the broiler element. Line a baking sheet with aluminum foil.
6. When the timer beeps, use a natural pressure release for 15 minutes and then release any remaining pressure. Carefully open the lid.
7. Transfer the ribs with tongs to the prepared baking sheet, meaty side up.
8. Stir the cooking liquid and pour over the ribs with a spoon. Broil the ribs for 5 minutes until browned in places.
9. Transfer the ribs to a serving plate and serve warm.

Indian Roasted Pork

Prep time: 6 mins, Cook Time: 8 hours, Servings: 3

- 1 tbsp. olive oil
- 1 lb. pork loin
- 1 tsp. cumin
- 2 garlic cloves, roughly chopped
- 1 onion, sliced
- Salt and pepper, to taste

1. Coat the Instant Pot with olive oil and add the pork loin. Set aside.
2. In a food processor, place the remaining ingredients.
3. Pulse until smooth then pour the mixture over the pork loin.
4. Lock the lid. Press the Slow Cook button and set the cooking time to 8 hours at High Pressure.
5. Once cooking is complete, perform a natural pressure release for 10 minutes, and then release any remaining pressure. Carefully open the lid.
6. Allow to cool for a few minutes. Remove them from the pot and serve warm.

Instant Pot Rib

Prep time: 6 mins, Cook Time: 8 hours, Servings: 3

- 1 rack baby back rib
- 1 tbsp. smoked paprika
- 2 tbsps. olive oil
- 1 tbsp. onion powder
- 1 tbsp. garlic powder
- Salt and pepper, to taste
- ½ cup water

1. Prepare a baking sheet. Lay on the ribs. Rub with paprika, olive oil, onion powder, garlic powder, salt, and pepper.
2. Place the well-coated rib in the Instant Pot. Pour in the water.
3. Lock the lid. Press the Slow Cook button and set the cooking time to 8 hours at High Pressure.
4. Once cooking is complete, perform a natural pressure release for 10 minutes, and then release any remaining pressure. Carefully open the lid.
5. Allow to cool for a few minutes. Remove the rib from the pot and serve warm.

Italian Pork Cutlets

Prep time: 6 mins, Cook Time: 20 mins, Servings: 6

- 4 tbsps. olive oil
- 6 pork cutlets
- Salt and pepper, to taste
- 1 tbsp. Italian herb mix
- 1½ cups water

1. In the Instant Pot, add all the ingredients. Stir to combine well.
2. Lock the lid. Press the Meat/Stew button and set the cooking time to 20 minutes at High Pressure.
3. Once cooking is complete, do a natural pressure release for 10 minutes, and then release any remaining pressure. Carefully open the lid.
4. Remove the meat and serve immediately.

Jamaican Pork Roast

Prep time: 10 minutes | Cook time: 55 minutes | Serves 6

¼ cup Jamaican jerk spice blend
¾ tablespoon olive oil
2 pounds (907 g) pork shoulder
¼ cup beef broth

1. Rub the jerk spice blend and olive oil all over the pork shoulder and set aside to marinate for 10 minutes.
2. When ready, press the Sauté button on the Instant Pot and add the pork.
3. Sear for 4 minutes. Flip the pork and cook for 4 minutes.
4. Pour the beef broth into the Instant Pot.
5. Secure the lid. Select the Manual mode and set the cooking time for 45 minutes at High Pressure.
6. Once cooking is complete, do a natural pressure release for 10 minutes, then release any remaining pressure. Carefully open the lid.
7. Serve hot.

Maple-Glazed Spareribs

Prep time: 40 minutes | Cook time: 30 minutes | Serves 6

2 racks (about 3 pounds / 1.4 kg) baby back pork ribs, cut into 2-rib sections
1 teaspoon instant coffee crystals
1 teaspoon sea salt
½ teaspoon ground cumin
½ teaspoon chili powder
½ teaspoon ground mustard
½ teaspoon cayenne pepper
½ teaspoon onion powder
½ teaspoon garlic powder
¼ teaspoon ground coriander
¼ cup soy sauce
¼ cup pure maple syrup
2 tablespoons tomato paste
1 tablespoon apple cider vinegar
1 tablespoon olive oil
1 medium onion, peeled and large diced

1. Mix together the coffee, salt, cumin, chili powder, mustard, cayenne pepper, onion powder, garlic powder, and coriander in a mixing bowl. Rub the mixture into the rib sections with your hands. Refrigerate for at least 30 minutes, covered. Set aside.
2. Stir together the soy sauce, maple syrup, tomato paste, and apple cider vinegar in a small mixing bowl.
3. Set your Instant Pot to Sauté and heat the olive oil. Add the onions and sauté for 3 to 5 minutes until translucent.
4. Stir in the soy sauce mixture. Add a few ribs at a time with tongs and gently stir to coat. Arrange the ribs standing upright, meat-side outward. Secure the lid.
5. Select the Manual function and cook for 25 minutes on High Pressure.
6. Once cooking is complete, use a natural pressure release for 10 minutes and then release any remaining pressure. Carefully open the lid.
7. Transfer the ribs to a serving plate and serve warm.

Mexican Chili Pork

Prep time: 6 mins, Cook Time: 35 mins, Servings: 6

- 3 tbsps. olive oil
- 2 tsps. minced garlic
- 2 lbs. pork sirloin, sliced
- 2 tsps. ground cumin
- 1 tbsp. red chili flakes
- 1 cup water
- Salt and pepper, to taste

1. Press the Sauté button on the Instant pot and heat the olive oil until shimmering.
2. Add and sauté the garlic for 30 seconds or until fragrant.
3. Add the pork sirloin and sauté for 3 minutes or until lightly browned.

4. Add the cumin and chili flakes.

5. Pour in the water and sprinkle salt and pepper for seasoning.

6. Lock the lid. Press the Meat/Stew button and set the cooking time to 30 minutes at High Pressure.

7. Once cooking is complete, perform a natural pressure release for 10 minutes, and then release any remaining pressure. Carefully open the lid.

8. Remove the pork from the pot and serve warm.

Pulled Pork

Prep time: 6 mins, Cook Time: 1 hour, Servings: 12

- 4 lbs. pork shoulder
- 1 tsp. cinnamon
- 2 tsps. garlic powder
- 5 tbsps. coconut oil
- 1 tsp. cumin powder
- 1½ cups water
- Salt and pepper, to taste

1. In the Instant Pot, add all the ingredients. Stir to combine well.

2. Lock the lid. Press the Meat/Stew button and set the cooking time to 1 hour at High Pressure.

3. Once cooking is complete, do a natural pressure release for 10 minutes, and then release any remaining pressure. Carefully open the lid.

4. Remove the meat and shred with two forks to serve.

Pork and Mushroom with Mustard

Prep time: 6 mins, Cook Time: 35 mins, Servings: 6

- 3 tbsps. butter
- 2 lbs. pork shoulder
- 3 tbsps. yellow mustard
- 1 cup water
- 1 cup sliced mushrooms
- Salt and pepper, to taste

1. Press the Sauté button on the Instant Pot and heat the butter until melted.

2. Add the pork shoulder and mustard. Sauté for 3 minutes or until the pork is lightly browned.

3. Stir in water and mushrooms. Sprinkle salt and pepper for seasoning.

4. Lock the lid. Press the Meat/Stew button and set the cooking time to 30 minutes at High Pressure.

5. Once cooking is complete, perform a natural pressure release for 10 minutes, and then release any remaining pressure. Carefully open the lid.

6. Remove the pork from the pot and serve warm.

Paprika Pork with Brussels Sprouts

Prep time: 10 minutes | Cook time: 30 minutes | Serves 4

2 tablespoons olive oil

2 pounds (907 g) pork shoulder, cubed

2 cups Brussels sprouts, trimmed and halved

1½ cups beef stock

1 tablespoon sweet paprika

1 tablespoon chopped parsley

1. Press the Sauté button on the Instant Pot and heat the olive oil.

2. Add the pork and brown for 5 minutes. Stir in the remaining ingredients.

3. Secure the lid. Select the Manual mode and set the cooking time for 25 minutes at High Pressure.

4. Once cooking is complete, do a natural pressure release for 10 minutes, then release any remaining pressure. Carefully open the lid.

5. Divide the mix between plates and serve warm.

Pork with Bell Peppers

Prep time: 10 minutes | Cook time: 35 minutes | Serves 4

2 tablespoons olive oil

4 pork chops

1 red onion, chopped

3 garlic cloves, minced

1 red bell pepper, roughly chopped

1 green bell pepper, roughly chopped

2 cups beef stock

A pinch of salt and black pepper

1 tablespoon parsley, chopped

1. Press the Sauté on your Instant Pot. Add and heat the oil. Brown the pork chops for 2 minutes.

2. Fold in the onion and garlic and brown for an additional 3 minutes.

3. Stir in the bell peppers, stock, salt, and pepper.

4. Lock the lid. Select the Manual mode and cook for 30 minutes on High Pressure.

5. Once cooking is complete, use a natural pressure release for 10 minutes and then release any remaining pressure. Carefully open the lid.

6. Divide the mix among the plates and serve topped with the parsley.

Pork with Brussels Sprouts

Prep time: 10 minutes | Cook time: 30 minutes | Serves 4

1½ pound (680 g) pork chops
1 pound (454 g) Brussels sprouts, trimmed and halved
2 tablespoons Cajun seasoning
1 cup beef stock
A pinch of salt and black pepper
1 tablespoon parsley, chopped

1. Stir together all the ingredients in your Instant Pot.

2. Secure the lid. Press the Manual button on the Instant Pot and set the cooking time for 30 minutes on High Pressure.

3. Once cooking is complete, perform a natural pressure release for 10 minutes and then release any remaining pressure. Carefully open the lid.

4. Divide the mix among the plates and serve immediately.

Pork Shoulder and Celery

Prep time: 10 minutes | Cook time: 30 minutes | Serves 4

2 tablespoons avocado oil
4 garlic cloves, minced
2 pounds (907 g) pork shoulder, boneless and cubed
1½ cups beef stock
2 celery stalks, chopped
2 tablespoons chili powder
1 tablespoon chopped sage
A pinch of salt and black pepper

1. Press the Sauté button on the Instant Pot and heat the avocado oil.

2. Add the garlic and sauté for 2 minutes until fragrant.

3. Stir in the pork and brown for another 3 minutes.

4. Add the remaining ingredients to the Instant Pot and mix well.

5. Secure the lid. Select the Manual mode and set the cooking time for 25 minutes at High Pressure.

6. Once cooking is complete, do a natural pressure release for 10 minutes, then release any remaining pressure. Carefully open the lid.

7. Serve warm.

Vinegary Pork Chops with Figs and Pears

Prep time: 10 minutes | Cook time: 10 minutes | Serves 2

2 (1-inch-thick) bone-in pork chops
1 teaspoon sea salt
1 teaspoon ground black pepper
¼ cup chicken broth
¼ cup balsamic vinegar
1 tablespoon dried mint
2 tablespoons avocado oil
5 dried figs, stems removed and halved
3 pears, peeled, cored, and diced large
1 medium sweet onion, peeled and sliced

1. Pat the pork chops dry with a paper towel and sprinkle both sides generously with the salt and pepper. Set aside.

2. Stir together the broth, vinegar, and mint in a small bowl. Set aside.

3. Set the Instant Pot to Sauté. Add and heat the oil. Sear the pork chops for 5 minutes on each side and transfer to a plate.

4. Pour in the broth mixture and deglaze the Instant Pot, scraping any browned bits from the pot.

5. Add the onions to the pot and scatter the figs and pears on top. Return the pork chops to the pot.

6. Secure the lid. Select the Steam function and cook for 3 minutes on High Pressure.

7. Once the timer goes off, do a natural pressure release for 10 minutes and then release any remaining pressure. Carefully open the lid.

8. Transfer to a serving dish with a slotted spoon. Serve immediately.

CHAPTER 8 LAMB

Black Bean Minced Lamb

Prep time: 10 minutes | Cook time: 25 minutes | Serves 4 to 6

1 pound (454 g) ground lamb
2 tablespoons vegetable oil
½ cup chopped onion
½ teaspoon salt
2 cans drained black beans
1 can undrained diced tomatoes
1 can chopped and undrained green chillies
1½ cups chicken broth
1½ tablespoons tomato paste
1½ tablespoons chili powder
2 teaspoons cumin
½ teaspoon cayenne

1. Set the Instant Pot to the Sauté mode and heat the oil. Add the lamb, onion and salt to the pot and sauté for 5 minutes, stirring constantly. Add the remaining ingredients to the pot and stir well.
2. Select the Manual setting and set the cooking time for 20 minutes on High Pressure. Once the timer goes off, use a natural pressure release for 10 minutes, then release any remaining pressure. Carefully open the lid.
3. Serve immediately.

Braised Lamb Ragout

Prep time: 10 minutes | Cook time: 1 hour 8 minutes | Serves 4 to 6

1½ pounds (680 g) lamb, bone-in
1 teaspoon vegetable oil
4 tomatoes, chopped
2 carrots, sliced
½ pound (227 g) mushrooms, sliced
1 small yellow onion, chopped
6 cloves garlic, minced
2 tablespoons tomato paste
1 teaspoon dried oregano
Water, as needed
Salt and ground black pepper, to taste
Handful chopped parsley

1. Press the Sauté button on the Instant Pot and heat the olive oil. Add the lamb and sear for 4 minutes per side, or until browned.
2. Stir in the tomatoes, carrots, mushrooms, onion, garlic, tomato paste, oregano and water. Season with salt and pepper.
3. Set the lid in place. Select the Manual mode and set the cooking time for 60 minutes on High Pressure. Once cooking is complete, perform a quick pressure release. Carefully open the lid.
4. Transfer the lamb to a plate. Discard the bones and shred the meat. Return the shredded lamb to the pot, add the parsley and stir.
5. Serve warm.

Lamb Curry

Prep time: 10 minutes | Cook time: 30 minutes | Serves 4

1 teaspoon curry paste
2 tablespoons coconut cream
¼ teaspoon chili powder
1 pound (454 g) lamb shoulder, chopped
1 tablespoon fresh cilantro, chopped
½ cup heavy cream

1. In a bowl, mix the curry paste and coconut cream.
2. Add the chili powder and chopped lamb shoulder. Toss to coat the lamb in the curry mixture well.
3. Transfer the lamb and all remaining curry paste mixture in the Instant Pot. Add cilantro and heavy cream.
4. Close the lid and select Manual mode. Set cooking time for 30 minutes on High Pressure.
5. When timer beeps, do a quick pressure release. Open the lid.
6. Serve warm.

Lamb Burgers

Prep time: 10 minutes | Cook time: 14 minutes | Serves 2

10 ounces (283 g) ground lamb
½ teaspoon chili powder
1 teaspoon dried cilantro
1 teaspoon garlic powder
½ teaspoon salt
¼ cup water
1 tablespoon coconut oil

1. In a mixing bowl, mix the ground lamb, chili powder, dried cilantro, garlic powder, salt, and water.
2. Shape the mixture into 2 burgers.
3. Melt the coconut oil on Sauté mode.
4. Put the burgers in the hot oil and cook for 7 minutes on each side or until well browned.
5. Serve immediately.

Garlicky Lamb Leg

Prep time: 35 minutes | Cook time: 50 minutes | Serves 6

2 pounds (907 g) lamb leg
6 garlic cloves, minced
1 teaspoon sea salt
1½ teaspoons black pepper
2½ tablespoons olive oil
1½ small onions
1½ cups bone broth
¾ cup orange juice
6 sprigs thyme

1. In a bowl, whisk together the garlic, salt and pepper. Add the lamb leg to the bowl and marinate for 30 minutes.
2. Press the Sauté button on the Instant Pot and heat the olive oil. Add the onions and sauté for 4 minutes. Transfer the onions to a separate bowl.
3. Add the marinated lamb to the pot and sear for 3 minutes on each side, or lightly browned. Whisk in the cooked onions, broth, orange juice and thyme.
4. Close and secure the lid. Set the Instant Pot to the Meat/Stew mode and set the cooking time for 40 minutes on High Pressure. When the timer beeps, use a natural pressure release for 10 minutes, then release any remaining pressure. Carefully open the lid.
5. Divide the dish among 6 serving bowls and serve hot.

Greek Lamb Leg

Prep time: 10 minutes | Cook time: 50 minutes | Serves 4

1 pound (454 g) lamb leg
½ teaspoon dried thyme
1 teaspoon paprika powder
¼ teaspoon cumin seeds
1 tablespoon softened butter
2 garlic cloves
¼ cup water

1. Rub the lamb leg with dried thyme, paprika powder, and cumin seeds on a clean work surface.
2. Brush the leg with softened butter and transfer to the Instant Pot. Add garlic cloves and water.
3. Close the lid. Select Manual mode and set cooking time for 50 minutes on High Pressure.
4. When timer beeps, use a quick pressure release. Open the lid.
5. Serve warm.

Greek Lamb Loaf

Prep time: 5 minutes | Cook time: 15 minutes | Serves 2

1 pound (454 g) ground lamb meat
4 garlic cloves
½ small onion, chopped
1 teaspoon ground marjoram
1 teaspoon rosemary
¾ teaspoon salt
¼ teaspoon black pepper
¾ cup water

1. In a blender, combine the lamb meat, garlic, onions, marjoram, rosemary, salt and pepper. Pulse until well mixed. Shape the lamb mixture into a compact loaf and cover tightly with aluminium foil. Use a fork to make some holes.

2. Pour the water into the Instant Pot and put a trivet in the pot. Place the lamb loaf on the trivet and lock the lid.

3. Select the Manual mode and set the cooking time for 15 minutes on High Pressure. When the timer goes off, use a quick pressure release.

4. Carefully open the lid. Serve warm.

Harissa Lamb

Prep time: 30 minutes | Cook time: 40 minutes | Serves 4

1 tablespoon keto-friendly Harissa sauce

1 teaspoon dried thyme

½ teaspoon salt

1 pound (454 g) lamb shoulder

2 tablespoons sesame oil

2 cups water

1. In a bowl, mix the Harissa, dried thyme, and salt.

2. Rub the lamb shoulder with the Harissa mixture and brush with sesame oil.

3. Heat the the Instant Pot on Sauté mode for 2 minutes and put the lamb shoulder inside.

4. Cook the lamb for 3 minutes on each side, then pour in the water.

5. Close the lid. Select Manual mode and set cooking time for 40 minutes on High Pressure.

6. When timer beeps, use a natural pressure release for 25 minutes, then release any remaining pressure. Open the lid.

7. Serve warm.

Herbed Lamb Shank

Prep time: 15 minutes | Cook time: 35 minutes | Serves 2

2 lamb shanks

1 rosemary spring

1 teaspoon coconut flour

¼ teaspoon onion powder

¼ teaspoon chili powder

¾ teaspoon ground ginger

½ cup beef broth

½ teaspoon avocado oil

1. Put all ingredients in the Instant Pot. Stir to mix well.

2. Close the lid. Select Manual mode and set cooking time for 35 minutes on High Pressure.

3. When timer beeps, use a natural pressure release for 15 minutes, then release any remaining pressure. Open the lid.

4. Discard the rosemary sprig and serve warm.

Icelandic Lamb with Turnip

Prep time: 5 minutes | Cook time: 45 minutes | Serves 4

12 ounces (340 g) lamb fillet, chopped

4 ounces (113 g) turnip, chopped

3 ounces (85 g) celery ribs, chopped

1 teaspoon unsweetened tomato purée

¼ cup scallions, chopped

½ teaspoon salt

½ teaspoon ground black pepper

4 cups water

1. Put all ingredients in the Instant Pot and stir well.

2. Close the lid. Select Manual mode and set cooking time for 45 minutes on High Pressure.

3. When timer beeps, use a quick pressure release. Open the lid.

4. Serve hot.

Indian Lamb Curry

Prep time: 15 minutes | Cook time: 1 hour 3 minutes | Serves 4

2 tablespoons olive oil

1 pound (454 g) lamb meat, cubed

2 tomatoes, chopped

1 onion, chopped

1-inch piece ginger, grated

2 garlic cloves, minced

½ tablespoon ground cumin

½ tablespoon chili flakes

½ tablespoon ground turmeric

½ teaspoon garam masala

1 cup chicken stock

½ cup coconut milk

¼ cup rice, rinsed

1 tablespoon fish sauce

¼ cup chopped cilantro

1. Set the Instant Pot on the Sauté mode. Heat the olive oil and sear the lamb shoulder on both sides for 8 minutes, or until browned. Transfer the lamb to a plate and set aside.

2. Add the tomatoes, onion, ginger and garlic to the pot and sauté for 5 minutes. Stir in the cumin, chili flakes, turmeric and garam masala. Cook for 10 minutes, or until they form a paste. Whisk in the chicken stock, coconut milk, rice and fish sauce. Return the lamb back to the pot.

3. Lock the lid. Select Meat/Stew mode and set the cooking time for 35 minutes on High Pressure. Once cooking is complete, do a natural pressure release for 10 minutes, then release any remaining pressure. Open the lid and select the Sauté mode. Cook the curry for 5 minutes, or until thickened.

4. Top with the chopped cilantro and serve warm in bowls.

Indian Lamb Korma

Prep time: 15 minutes | Cook time: 25 minutes | Serves 6

1 (6-inch) Anaheim chile, minced

1 clove garlic, grated

½ medium onion, chopped

2 tablespoons coconut oil

½ teaspoon grated fresh ginger

1 teaspoon garam masala

¼ teaspoon ground cardamom

Pinch of ground cinnamon

2 teaspoons ground cumin

1 teaspoon coriander seeds

1 teaspoon sea salt

½ teaspoon cayenne pepper

½ tablespoon unsweetened tomato purée

1 cup chicken broth

3 pounds (1.4 kg) lamb shoulder, cut into 1-inch cubes

¼ cup full-fat coconut milk

½ cup full-fat Greek yogurt

1. Preheat the Instant Pot on Sauté mode. Add the chile, garlic, onion, coconut oil, and ginger and sauté for 2 minutes.

2. Add the garam masala, cardamom, cinnamon, cumin, coriander seeds, salt, cayenne, and unsweetened tomato purée and sauté for a minute or until fragrant.

3. Pour in the broth. Add the lamb and stir well.

4. Secure the lid. Press the Manual button and set cooking time for 15 minutes on High Pressure.

5. When timer beeps, quick release the pressure. Open the lid.

6. Stir in the coconut milk and yogurt. Switch to Sauté mode and bring the mixture to a simmer for 5 minutes, stirring occasionally until thickened.

7. Serve hot.

Lamb Meatballs

Prep time: 10 minutes | Cook time: 38 minutes | Serves 3

¾ pound (340 g) ground lamb meat

1 teaspoon adobo seasoning

½ tablespoon olive oil

2 small tomatoes, chopped roughly

5 mini bell peppers, deseeded and halved

2 garlic cloves, peeled

½ small yellow onion, chopped roughly

½ cup sugar-free tomato sauce

¼ teaspoon crushed red pepper flakes,

Salt and freshly ground black pepper, to taste

1. Mix the lamb meat and adobo seasoning in a bowl until well combined. Shape the meat mixture into small meatballs.

2. Set the Instant Pot on the Sauté mode and heat the olive oil. Add the meatballs to the pot and cook for 3 minutes, or until golden brown. Transfer the meatballs to bowls.

3. Stir together all the remaining ingredients in the pot. Lock the lid. Select the Meat/Stew mode and set the cooking time for 35 minutes on High Pressure. When the timer beeps, use a natural pressure release for 10 minutes, then release any remaining pressure.

4. Carefully open the lid. Transfer the vegetable mixture to a blender and pulse until smooth. Spread the vegetable paste over the meatballs and serve hot.

Lamb and Tomato Bhuna

Prep time: 15 minutes | Cook time: 20 minutes | Serves 2

¼ teaspoon minced ginger

¼ teaspoon garlic paste

1 teaspoon coconut oil

¼ cup crushed tomatoes

10 ounces (283 g) lamb fillet, chopped

2 ounces (57 g) scallions, chopped

¼ cup water

1. Put the minced ginger, garlic paste, coconut oil, and crushed tomatoes in the Instant Pot. Sauté for 10 minutes on Sauté mode.
2. Add the chopped lamb fillet, scallions, and water.
3. Select Manual mode and set cooking time for 10 minutes on High Pressure.
4. When timer beeps, use a natural pressure release for 15 minutes, then release any remaining pressure. Open the lid.
5. Serve warm.

Lamb Curry with Tomatoes

Prep time: 15 minutes | Cook time: 59 minutes | Serves 4

¼ cup olive oil, divided

2 pounds (907 g) lamb shoulder, cubed

4 green onions, sliced

2 tomatoes, peeled and chopped

2 tablespoons garlic paste

1 tablespoon ginger paste

1½ cups vegetable stock

2 teaspoons ground coriander

2 teaspoons allspice

1 teaspoon ground cumin

½ teaspoon ground red chili pepper

½ teaspoon curry powder

1 large carrot, sliced

1 potato, cubed

2 bay leaves

Salt, to taste

2 tablespoons mint leaves, chopped

1. Press the Sauté button on the Instant Pot and heat 2 tablespoons of the olive oil. Add the green onions and sauté for 3 minutes, or until softened, stirring constantly. Transfer the green onions to a blender. Mix in the tomatoes, garlic paste and ginger paste. Blend until smooth.
2. Heat the remaining 2 tablespoons of the olive oil in the pot and add the lamb to the pot. Cook for 6 minutes. Stir in the vegetable stock, coriander, allspice, cumin, red chili pepper, curry powder, carrot, potato, bay leaves and salt.
3. Lock the lid. Select the Manual function and set the cooking time for 50 minutes on High Pressure. When the timer beeps, use a natural pressure release for 10 minutes, then release any remaining pressure. Open the lid. Discard the bay leaves.
4. Top with the mint leaves and serve immediately.

Roasted Lamb Leg

Prep time: 10 minutes | Cook time: 25 minutes | Serves 3

14 ounces (397 g) lamb leg, roughly chopped

1 teaspoon dried thyme

1 teaspoon ground black pepper

1 tablespoon sesame oil

¼ cup beef broth

½ cup water

1. Rub the lamb leg with thyme, ground black pepper, and sesame oil on a clean work surface.
2. Put the leg in the Instant Pot, add beef broth and water.
3. Close the lid. Select Manual mode and set cooking time for 25 minutes on High Pressure.
4. When timer beeps, make a quick pressure release. Open the lid.
5. Serve warm.

Slow Cooked Lamb Shanks

Prep time: 10 minutes | Cook time: 55 minutes | Serves 4

2 tablespoons olive oil
2 pounds (907 g) lamb shanks
Salt and black pepper, to taste
6 garlic cloves, minced
1 cup chicken broth
¾ cup red wine
2 cups crushed tomatoes
1 teaspoon dried oregano
¼ cup chopped parsley, for garnish

1. Press the Sauté button on the Instant Pot. Heat the olive oil and add the lamb to the pot. Season with salt and pepper. Sear the lamb on both sides for 6 minutes, or until browned. Transfer the lamb to a plate and set aside.
2. Add the garlic to the pot and sauté for 30 seconds, or until fragrant. Stir in the chicken broth and red wine and cook for 2 minutes, stirring constantly. Add the tomatoes and oregano. Stir and cook for 2 minutes. Return the lamb to the pot and baste with the chicken broth mixture.
3. Lock the lid. Select the Manual setting and set the cooking time for 45 minutes on High Pressure.
4. When the timer beeps, do a natural pressure release for 15 minutes, then release any remaining pressure. Open the lid. Top with the chopped parsley and adjust the taste with salt and pepper.
5. Divide among 4 plates and serve warm.

Spicy Lamb Shoulder

Prep time: 10 minutes | Cook time: 50 minutes | Serves 4

2 pounds (907 g) lamb shoulder
1 cup chopped fresh thyme
¼ cup rice wine
¼ cup chicken stock
1 tablespoon turmeric
1 tablespoon ground black pepper
1 teaspoon oregano
1 teaspoon paprika
1 teaspoon sugar
1 tablespoon olive oil
½ cup water
4 tablespoons butter

1. In a large bowl, whisk together the thyme, rice wine, chicken stock, turmeric, black pepper, oregano, paprika and sugar. Rub all sides of the lamb shoulder with the spice mix.
2. Press the Sauté button on the Instant Pot and heat the oil. Add the lamb to the pot and sear for 5 minutes on both sides, or until browned. Add the remaining spice mixture, water and butter to the pot. Stir until the butter is melted.
3. Lock the lid. Select the Manual mode and set the cooking time for 45 minutes on High Pressure. Once cooking is complete, do a natural pressure release for 10 minutes, then release any remaining pressure. Carefully open the lid.
4. Serve hot.

Lamb with Anchovies

Prep time: 10 minutes | Cook time: 1 hour 5 minutes | Serves 4

2 tablespoons olive oil
2 pounds (907 g) boneless lamb shoulder, cut into 4 pieces
2 cups chicken stock
6 tinned anchovies, chopped
1 teaspoon garlic purée
3 green chilies, minced
1 sprig rosemary
1 teaspoon dried oregano
Salt, to taste
2 tablespoons chopped parsley

1. Press the Sauté button on the Instant Pot. Heat the olive oil and sear the lamb shoulder on both sides for 5 minutes, or until browned. Transfer the lamb to a plate and set aside.
2. Pour the chicken stock into the Instant Pot and add the anchovies and garlic. Return the lamb to the pot and sprinkle the green chilies, rosemary, oregano and salt on top.

3. Set the lid in place, select the Manual mode and set the cooking time for 60 minutes on High Pressure.
4. When the timer goes off, use a natural pressure release for 15 minutes, then release any remaining pressure.
5. Open the lid, shred the lamb with two forks and top with the chopped parsley. Serve warm.

Spicy Minced Lamb Meat

Prep time: 10 minutes | Cook time: 20 minutes | Serves 2

½ pound (227 g) ground lamb meat
½ cup onion, chopped
½ tablespoon minced ginger
½ tablespoon garlic
½ teaspoon salt
¼ teaspoon ground coriander
¼ teaspoon cayenne pepper
¼ teaspoon cumin
¼ teaspoon turmeric

1. Press the Sauté button on the Instant Pot. Add the onion, ginger and garlic to the pot and sauté for 5 minutes. Add the remaining ingredients to the pot and lock the lid.
2. Select the Manual mode and set the cooking time for 15 minutes on High Pressure. Once the timer goes off, perform a natural pressure release for 15 minutes.
3. Open the lid and serve immediately.

Lamb Casserole

Prep time: 15 minutes | Cook time: 41 minutes | Serves 2 to 4

1 pound (454 g) lamb stew meat, cubed
1 tablespoon olive oil
3 cloves garlic, minced
2 tomatoes, chopped
2 carrots, chopped
1 onion, chopped
1 pound (454 g) baby potatoes
1 celery stalk, chopped
2 cups chicken stock
2 tablespoons red wine

2 tablespoons ketchup
1 teaspoon ground cumin
1 teaspoon sweet paprika
¼ teaspoon dried rosemary
¼ teaspoon dried oregano
Salt and ground black pepper, to taste

1. Press the Sauté button on the Instant Pot and heat the oil. Add the lamb to the pot and sear for 5 minutes, or until lightly browned. Add the garlic and sauté for 1 minute. Add all the remaining ingredients to the pot.
2. Set the lid in place. Select the Manual mode and set the cooking time for 35 minutes on High Pressure. Once cooking is complete, perform a natural pressure release for 10 minutes, then release any remaining pressure. Carefully open the lid.
3. Serve hot.

Lamb Rogan Josh

Prep time: 15 minutes | Cook time: 35 to 37 minutes | Serves 4

2 tablespoons ghee
1 large onion, chopped
2 pounds (907 g) boneless lamb shoulder, cubed
4 teaspoons chili powder
3 teaspoons coriander powder
2 teaspoons minced ginger
1 teaspoon garam masala
1 teaspoon turmeric
½ teaspoon cinnamon powder
½ teaspoon cardamom powder
¼ teaspoon ground cloves
¼ teaspoon cumin powder
10 garlic cloves, minced
1 bay leaf
Salt and black pepper, to taste
1 (15-ounce / 425-g) can tomato sauce
8 tablespoons plain yogurt
1 cup water
3 tablespoons chopped cilantro

1. Select the Sauté mode. Melt the ghee and add the onion and lamb to the pot. Cook for 6 to 7 minutes, or until the lamb is lightly browned.

2.   Add the chili powder, coriander, ginger, garam masala, turmeric, cinnamon, cardamom, cloves, cumin, garlic, bay leaf, salt and pepper to the pot. Cook for 3 minutes, or until fragrant.

3.   Stir in the tomato sauce and cook for 2 to 3 minutes. Add the yogurt, 1 tablespoon at a time, stirring to combine. Pour the water in the pot.

4.   Lock the lid. Select Manual mode and set the cooking time for 20 minutes on High Pressure.

5.   When the timer goes off, do a natural pressure release for 10 minutes, then release any remaining pressure. Open the lid and select the Sauté mode. Cook for another 4 minutes to boil off some liquid until the consistency is stew-like.

6.   Divide the dish among 4 bowls. Top with the chopped cilantro and serve warm.

CHAPTER 9 PASTA AND RICE

Beef and Cheddar Pasta

Prep time: 5 minutes | Cook time: 12 to 13 minutes | Serves 4 to 6

1 teaspoon olive oil

1¼ pound (567 g) ground beef

1 packet onion soup mix

3½ cups hot water

3 beef bouillon cubes

1 pound (454 g) elbow macaroni

8 ounces (227 g) sharp Cheddar cheese, grated

Salt and ground black pepper, to taste

1. Press the Sauté button on your Instant Pot. Pour in the oil and let heat for 1 minute.
2. Add the ground beef and sauté for 4 to 5 minutes until browned.
3. Mix together the onion soup mix, water, and bouillon cubes in a bowl.
4. Add the mixture and macaroni to the pot and stir to combine.
5. Press the Manual button on your Instant Pot and cook for 7 minutes at High Pressure.
6. When the timer goes off, perform a quick pressure release. Carefully open the lid.
7. Stir in the Cheddar cheese and let stand for 5 minutes.
8. Taste and sprinkle with salt and pepper if needed.
9. Serve.

Pizza Pasta

Prep time: 5 minutes | Cook time: 5 to 8 minutes | Serves 6

4 cups of noodles such as ziti or riganoti

8 cups of water

2 cups of spaghetti sauce

1½ cup of shredded mozzarella cheese

10 pepperoni, cut in half

1. Add the noodles and water to the Instant Pot.
2. Lock the lid. Press the Manual button on the Instant Pot and cook for 3 minutes at High Pressure.

3. Once cooking is complete, perform a quick pressure release. Carefully remove the lid. Drain the cooking liquid.
4. Return the pasta to the Instant Pot. Fold in the spaghetti sauce, shredded cheese, and sliced pepperoni. Stir well.
5. Press the Sauté button on the Instant Pot. Cook for 2 to 3 minutes, or until the sauce starts to bubble and the cheese has melted, stirring occasionally.
6. Serve immediately.

Turkey Spaghetti

Prep time: 10 minutes | Cook time: 16 minutes | Serves 4 to 6

1 teaspoon olive oil

1 pound (454 g) ground turkey

1 clove garlic, minced

¼ onion, diced

8 ounces (227 g) whole wheat spaghetti, halved

1 jar (25-ounce / 709-g) Delallo Pomodoro Tomato-Basil Sauce (or of your choice)

¾ teaspoon kosher salt

2 cups water

shredded Parmesan cheese (optional)

1. Set your Instant Pot to Sauté. Add and heat the oil.
2. Add the ground turkey and sauté for 3 minutes.
3. Fold in the garlic and onion. Sauté for another 4 minutes.
4. Mix in the spaghetti, sauce and salt. Add the water to the pot and stir to combine.
5. Secure the lid. Press the Manual button on the Instant Pot and cook for 9 minutes on High Pressure.
6. Once the cooking is complete, do a quick pressure release. Carefully remove the lid.
7. Serve topped with the shredded cheese.

Broccoli and Chicken Rice

Prep time: 5 minutes | Cook time: 20 minutes | Serves 4 to 6

2 tablespoons butter
2 cloves garlic, minced
1 onion, chopped
1½ pounds (680 g) boneless chicken breasts, sliced
Salt and ground black pepper, to taste
1⅓ cups chicken broth
1⅓ cups long grain rice
½ cup milk
1 cup broccoli florets
½ cup grated Cheddar cheese

1. Set your Instant Pot to Sauté and melt the butter.
2. Add the garlic, onion, and chicken pieces to the pot. Season with salt and pepper to taste.
3. Sauté for 5 minutes, stirring occasionally, or until the chicken is lightly browned.
4. Stir in the chicken broth, rice, milk, broccoli, and cheese.
5. Lock the lid. Select the Manual mode and set the cooking time for 15 minutes at High Pressure.
6. When the timer beeps, perform a natural pressure release for 10 minutes, then release any remaining pressure. Carefully remove the lid.
7. Divide into bowls and serve.

Chicken Fettuccine Alfredo

Prep time: 5 minutes | Cook time: 3 minutes | Serves 2

8 ounces (227 g) fettuccine, halved
2 cups water
2 teaspoons chicken seasoning
1 cup cooked and diced chicken
1 jar (15-ounce / 425-g) Alfredo sauce
Salt and ground black pepper, to taste

1. Add the pasta, water, and chicken seasoning to the Instant Pot and stir to combine.
2. Secure the lid. Press the Manual button on the Instant Pot and set the cooking time for 3 minutes at High Pressure.

3. When the timer goes off, perform a quick pressure release. Carefully remove the lid.
4. Drain the pasta and transfer to a serving bowl.
5. Add the cooked chicken and drizzle the sauce over the top. Sprinkle with salt and pepper.
6. Stir until well mixed and serve.

Tomato and Chickpea Rice

Prep time: 12 mins, Cook Time:25 mins, Servings: 4

- ½ cup canned chickpeas
- 4½ cups water
- 1 cup deseeded and minced ripe tomato
- Salt and pepper, to taste
- 2 cups rinsed and drained white rice

1. Pour all the ingredients into Instant Pot. Gently stir.
2. Lock the lid. Select the Rice mode, then set the timer for 5 minutes at Low Pressure.
3. Once the timer goes off, do a quick pressure release. Carefully open the lid.
4. Using a rice paddle, fluff up rice.
5. Serve immediately.

Chipotle Cilantro Rice

Prep time: 20 mins, Cook Time: 20 mins, Servings: 4

- 2 cups brown rice, rinsed
- 4 small bay leaves
- 2¾ cups water
- 1½ tbsps. olive oil
- ½ cup chopped cilantro
- 1 lime, juiced
- 1 tsp. salt

1. Place the brown rice, bay leaves, and water in the Instant Pot.
2. Lock the lid. Select the Rice mode and cook for 20 minutes at High Pressure.
3. Once cooking is complete, do a natural pressure release for 10 minutes, then release any remaining pressure. Carefully open the lid.
4. Add the olive oil, cilantro, lime juice, and salt to the pot and stir until well combined. Serve warm.

Cinnamon Brown Rice

Prep time: 5 minutes | Cook time: 25 minutes | Serves 4

1 tablespoon olive oil

3 cloves garlic, crushed and minced

½ cup chopped sweet yellow onion

½ teaspoon cumin

½ teaspoon nutmeg

½ teaspoon cinnamon

½ teaspoon sweet paprika

½ teaspoon sea salt

1½ cups brown rice

2½ cups vegetable broth

½ cup chopped fresh parsley

1. Set your Instant Pot to Sauté and heat the olive oil.

2. Add the garlic, onion, cumin, nutmeg, cinnamon, sweet paprika, and sea salt and sauté for 2 to 3 minutes, stirring frequently, or until the onions are softened.

3. Add the rice and vegetable broth to the Instant Pot.

4. Secure the lid. Select the Manual mode and set the cooking time for 20 minutes at High Pressure.

5. Once cooking is complete, do a quick pressure release. Carefully open the lid.

6. Fluff the rice with a fork and stir in the fresh parsley before serving.

Confetti Rice

Prep time: 5 minutes | Cook time: 12 minutes | Serves 4

3 tablespoons butter

1 small onion, chopped

1 cup long-grain white rice

3 cups frozen peas, thawed

1 cup vegetable broth

¼ cup lemon juice

2 cloves garlic, minced

1 tablespoon cumin powder

½ teaspoon salt

½ teaspoon black pepper

1. Set your Instant Pot to Sauté and melt the butter.

2. Add the onion and sauté for 3 minutes until soft. Add the remaining ingredients to the Instant Pot, stirring well.

3. Secure the lid. Select the Manual mode and set the cooking time for 8 minutes at High Pressure.

4. Once cooking is complete, do a quick pressure release. Carefully open the lid.

5. Fluff the rice and serve hot.

Cilantro Lime Rice

Prep time: 3 minutes; Cook Time: 10 mins, Servings: 2

*   1¼ cups water
*   1 cup white rice
*   Salt, to taste
*   3 tbsps. fresh chopped cilantro
*   1 tbsp. fresh lime juice
*   2 tbsps. vegetable oil

1. Mix the rice and water together in the Instant Pot and stir to combine. Season with salt.

2. Lock the lid. Select the Rice mode, then set the timer for 5 minutes at Low Pressure.

3. Once the timer goes off, do a natural pressure release for 3 to 5 minutes. Carefully open the lid.

4. Use a quick release to get rid of the remaining pressure. Use a fork to fluff up the rice.

5. Mix the lime juice, cilantro, and oil in a bowl.

6. Whisk well and mix into the rice. Serve immediately.

Broccoli Fettucine Pasta

Prep time: 10 minutes | Cook time: 8 to 9 minutes | Serves 8

1 teaspoon olive oil

3 garlic cloves, minced

2 cups minced broccoli

4¼ cups water, divided

1 pound (454 g) fettucine pasta

1 tablespoon butter

Salt, to taste

1 cup heavy cream

½ cup shredded Parmesan cheese

Ground black pepper, to taste

2 tablespoons minced parsley

1. Press the Sauté button on the Instant Pot and heat the oil. Add the garlic to the pot and sauté for 1 minute,

or until fragrant. Stir in the broccoli and ¼ cup of the water.

2. Set the lid in place. Select the Manual mode and set the cooking time for 3 minutes on High Pressure. When the timer goes off, do a quick pressure release. Carefully open the lid.

3. Drain the broccoli and transfer to a bowl.

4. Add the remaining 4 cups of the water, pasta, butter and salt to the Instant Pot and stir to combine.

5. Set the lid in place. Select the Manual mode and set the cooking time for 3 minutes on High Pressure. When the timer goes off, do a quick pressure release. Carefully open the lid. Drain any excess liquid from the pot.

6. Select the Sauté mode and stir in the cooked broccoli, heavy cream, Parmesan, salt and black pepper. Cook for 1 to 2 minutes.

7. Serve garnished with the parsley.

Kimchi Pasta

Prep time: 5 minutes | Cook time: 4 to 5 minutes | Serves 4 to 6
8 ounces (227 g) dried small pasta
2⅓ cups vegetable stock
2 garlic cloves, minced
½ red onion, sliced
½ to 1 teaspoon salt
1¼ cups kimchi, with any larger pieces chopped
½ cup coconut cream

1. In the Instant Pot, combine the pasta, stock, garlic, red onion and salt.

2. Set the lid in place. Select the Manual mode and set the cooking time for 1 minute on High Pressure. When the timer goes off, do a quick pressure release. Carefully open the lid.

3. Select Sauté mode. Stir in the kimchi. Simmer for 3 to 4 minutes. Stir in the coconut cream and serve.

Marsala Tofu Pasta

Prep time: 5 minutes | Cook time: 15 minutes | Serves 2
1 tablespoon butter
2 cups sliced mushrooms
1 small onion, diced
½ cup sun-dried tomatoes
½ cup tofu, diced into chunks
½ teaspoon garlic powder
1 cup white Marsala wine
1½ cups vegetable broth
1 cup Pennette pasta
½ cup grated goat cheese
¼ cup cream

1. Press the Sauté button on the Instant Pot and melt the butter. Add the mushrooms and onion to the pot and cook for 4 minutes. Add the tomatoes and tofu and cook for 3 minutes.

2. Add the garlic powder and cook for 1 minute. Pour in the white wine and cook for 1 minute. Stir in the broth. Add the pasta and don't stir.

3. Set the lid in place. Select the Manual mode and set the cooking time for 6 minutes on High Pressure. When the timer goes off, do a quick pressure release. Carefully open the lid.

4. Add the cheese and cream and let sit for 5 minutes. Serve hot.

Mushroom Alfredo Rice

Prep time: 5 minutes | Cook time: 25 minutes | Serves 4
2 tablespoons olive oil
¾ cup finely chopped onion
2 garlic cloves, minced
1 cup rice
2¾ cups vegetable broth
1½ tablespoons fresh lemon juice
Salt and black pepper, to taste
2 ounces (57 g) creamy mushroom Alfredo sauce
¼ cup coarsely chopped walnuts

1. Set your Instant Pot to Sauté. Add the oil, onion, and garlic to the pot and sauté for 3 minutes. Stir in the rice and broth.

2. Secure the lid. Select the Manual mode and set the cooking time for 22 minutes at High Pressure.

3. Once cooking is complete, do a natural pressure release for 10 minutes, then release any remaining pressure. Carefully open the lid.

4. Add lemon juice, salt, pepper, and sauce and stir to combine. Garnish with the chopped walnuts and serve.

Creamy Tomato Pasta with Spinach

Prep time: 5 minutes   Cook time: 9 minutes | Serves 4

1 (28-ounce / 794-g) can crushed tomatoes

10 ounces (284 g) penne, rotini, or fusilli (about 3 cups)

1 tablespoon dried basil

½ teaspoon garlic powder

½ teaspoon salt, plus more as needed

1½ cups water

1 cup unsweetened coconut milk

2 cups chopped fresh spinach (optional)

Freshly ground black pepper, to taste

1. Combine the tomatoes, pasta, basil, garlic powder, salt, and water in the Instant Pot.

2. Secure the lid. Select the Manual mode and set the cooking time for 4 minutes at High Pressure.

3. Once cooking is complete, do a natural pressure release for 5 minutes, then release any remaining pressure. Carefully open the lid.

4. Stir in the milk and spinach (if desired). Taste and season with more salt and pepper, as needed.

5. Set your Instant Pot to Sauté and let cook for 4 to 5 minutes, or until the sauce is thickened and the greens are wilt. Serve warm.

Spinach and Pine Nut Fusilli Pasta

Prep time: 5 minutes | Cook time: 12 minutes | Serves 4

1 tablespoon butter

2 garlic cloves, crushed

1 pound (454 g) spinach

1 pound (454 g) fusilli pasta

Salt and black pepper, to taste

Water, as needed

2 garlic cloves, chopped

¼ cup chopped pine nuts

Grated cheese, for serving

1. Press the Sauté button on the Instant Pot and melt the butter. Add the crushed garlic and spinach to the pot and sauté for 6 minutes. Add the pasta, salt and pepper. Pour in the water to cover the pasta and mix.

2. Set the lid in place. Select the Manual mode and set the cooking time for 6 minutes on Low Pressure. When the timer goes off, do a quick pressure release. Carefully open the lid.

3. Stir in the chopped garlic and nuts. Garnish with the cheese and serve.

Green Tea Risotto

Prep time: 6 mins, Cook Time: 20 mins, Servings: 4

- ¼ cup lentils, rinsed
- Salt, to taste
- 3 green tea bags
- 1 cup brown rice, rinsed
- 7 cups water

1. In the Instant Pot, add all ingredients and stir gently.

2. Lock the lid. Select the Manual mode, then set the timer for 20 minutes at Low Pressure.

3. Once the timer goes off, do a quick pressure release. Carefully open the lid.

4. Serve immediately.

Ground Beef Pasta

Prep time: 5 minutes | Cook time: 11 to 13 minutes | Serves 4

1 teaspoon olive oil

1 pound (454 g) ground beef

8 ounces (227 g) dried pasta

24 ounces (680 g) pasta sauce

1½ cup water

Salt and ground black pepper, to taste

Italian seasoning, to taste

1. Press the Sauté button on the Instant Pot. Add the oil and let heat for 1 minute.

2. Fold in the ground beef and cook for 3 to 5 minutes until browned, stirring frequently.

3. Mix in the pasta, sauce and water and stir to combine.

4. Secure the lid. Press the Manual button on the Instant Pot and set the cooking time for 7 minutes on High Pressure.

5. Once cooking is complete, do a quick pressure release. Carefully remove the lid.

6. Stir in salt, pepper, and Italian seasoning and stir well.

7. Transfer to a serving dish and serve immediately.

Pasta Carbonara

Prep time: 10 minutes | Cook time: 8 to 9 minutes | Serves 4

1 pound (454 g) pasta dry such as rigatoni, penne or cavatappi)
4 cups water
¼ teaspoon kosher salt
4 large eggs
1 cup grated Parmesan cheese
Ground black pepper, to taste
8 ounces (227 g) bacon pancetta or guanciale
4 tablespoons heavy cream

1.   Place the pasta, water, and salt in your Instant Pot.
2.   Secure the lid. Press the Manual button and cook for 5 minutes at High Pressure.
3.   Meantime, beat together the eggs, cheese and black pepper in a mixing bowl until well mixed.
4.   Cook the bacon on medium heat in a frying pan for 3 minutes until crispy.
5.   Once cooking is complete, do a quick pressure release. Carefully remove the lid.
6.   Select the Sauté mode. Transfer the bacon to the pot and cook for 30 seconds.
7.   Stir in the egg mixture and heavy cream.
8.   Secure the lid and let stand for 5 minutes.
9.   Transfer to a serving dish and serve.

Instant Pot Jasmine Rice

Prep time: 5 minutes | Cook time: 4 minutes | Serves 4 to 6

2 cups jasmine rice, rinsed
2 teaspoons olive oil
½ teaspoon salt
2 cups water

1.   Place all the ingredients into the Instant Pot and give a good stir.
2.   Lock the lid. Select the Manual mode and set the cooking time for 4 minutes at High Pressure.
3.   Once cooking is complete, do a natural pressure release for 10 minutes, then release any remaining pressure. Remove the lid.

4.   Fluff the rice with a fork and serve.

Cauliflower and Pineapple Jasmine Rice Bowl

Prep time: 5 minutes | Cook time: 20 minutes | Serves 4 to 6

4 cups water
2 cups jasmine rice
1 cauliflower, florets separated and chopped
½ pineapple, peeled and chopped
2 teaspoons extra virgin olive oil
Salt and ground black pepper, to taste

1.   Stir together all the ingredients in the Instant Pot.
2.   Lock the lid. Select the Manual mode and set the cooking time for 20 minutes at Low Pressure.
3.   When the timer beeps, perform a natural pressure release for 10 minutes, then release any remaining pressure. Carefully remove the lid.
4.   Fluff with the rice spatula or fork, then serve.

Jollof Rice

Prep time: 10 minutes | Cook time: 22 minutes | Serves 4

1 tablespoon corn oil
2 dried bay leaves
1 onion, finely chopped
2 garlic cloves, finely chopped
1 teaspoon finely chopped fresh ginger
1 jalapeño, seeded and finely chopped
2 tomatoes, coarsely chopped
2 tablespoons tomato paste
1½ teaspoons kosher salt
1 teaspoon paprika
½ teaspoon curry powder
1 cup chopped carrots
1 cup cauliflower florets (7 or 8 florets)
1 cup short-grain white rice, rinsed
2 cups water

1.   Press the Sauté button on the Instant Pot and heat the oil.

2. Once hot, add the bay leaves, onion, garlic, ginger, and jalapeños, and sauté for 5 minutes, or until the onion is translucent.

3. Stir in the tomatoes, tomato paste, and salt. Loosely place the lid on top, and cook for 3 minutes, or until the tomatoes are softened. Mix in the paprika and curry powder, then stir in the carrots and cauliflower. Add the rice and water and stir well.

4. Secure the lid. Select the Rice mode and set the cooking time for 12 minutes at Low Pressure.

5. Once cooking is complete, do a natural pressure release for 10 minutes, then release any remaining pressure. Carefully open the lid.

6. Let the rice cool for 15 minutes. Remove the bay leaves. Using a fork, gently fluff the rice and serve hot.

Bow Tie Pasta

Prep time: 5 minutes | Cook time: 11 to 12 minutes | Serves 4 to 5

1 Vidalia onion, diced
2 garlic cloves, minced
1 tablespoon olive oil
3½ cups water
10 ounces (284 g) bow tie pasta
Grated zest and juice of 1 lemon
¼ cup black olives, pitted and chopped
Salt and freshly ground black pepper, to taste

1. Press the Sauté button on the Instant Pot and heat the oil. Add the onion and garlic to the pot. Cook for 7 to 8 minutes, stirring occasionally, or until the onion is lightly browned.

2. Add the water and pasta.

3. Set the lid in place. Select the Manual mode and set the cooking time for 4 minutes on High Pressure. When the timer goes off, do a quick pressure release. Carefully open the lid.

4. Stir the pasta and drain any excess water. Stir in the lemon zest and juice and the olives. Season with salt and pepper.

5. Serve immediately.

Parmesan Pea Risotto

Prep time: 10 minutes | Cook time: 15 minutes | Serves 4

1 tablespoon extra-virgin olive oil
2 tablespoons butter, divided
1 yellow onion, chopped
1½ cups Arborio rice
2 tablespoons lemon juice
3½ cups chicken stock, divided
1½ cups frozen peas, thawed
2 tablespoons parsley, finely chopped
2 tablespoons parmesan, finely grated
1 teaspoon grated lemon zest
Salt and ground black pepper, to taste

1. Press the Sauté button on your Instant Pot. Add and heat the oil and 1 tablespoon of butter.

2. Add the onion and cook for 5 minutes, stirring occasionally. Mix in the rice and cook for an additional 3 minutes, stirring occasionally.

3. Stir in the lemon juice and 3 cups of stock.

4. Lock the lid. Select the Manual function and set the cooking time for 5 minutes at High Pressure.

5. Once cooking is complete, do a quick pressure release. Carefully open the lid.

6. Select the Sauté function again. Fold in the remaining ½ cup of stock and the peas and sauté for 2 minutes.

7. Add the remaining 1 tablespoon of butter, parsley, parmesan, lemon zest, salt, and pepper and stir well.

8. Serve.

Spinach Lemon Pasta

Prep time: 5 minutes | Cook time: 4 minutes | Serves 6

1 pound (454 g) fusilli pasta
4 cups chopped fresh spinach
4 cups vegetable broth
2 cloves garlic, crushed and minced
1 cup plain coconut milk
1 teaspoon lemon zest
1 teaspoon lemon juice
¼ cup chopped fresh parsley
1 tablespoon chopped fresh mint
½ teaspoon sea salt
½ teaspoon coarse ground black pepper

1. Stir together the fusilli pasta, spinach, vegetable broth and garlic in the Instant Pot.
2. Set the lid in place. Select the Manual mode and set the cooking time for 4 minutes on High Pressure.
3. Meanwhile, whisk together the coconut milk, lemon zest and lemon juice in a bowl.
4. When the timer goes off, do a quick pressure release. Carefully open the lid. Drain off any excess liquid that might remain.
5. Add the coconut milk mixture to the pasta, along with the parsley and mint. Season with salt and pepper.
6. Stir gently and let sit for 5 minutes before serving.

Duo-Cheese Mushroom Pasta

Prep time: 10 minutes | Cook time: 5 minutes | Serves 4

2 tablespoons butter
3 cloves garlic, minced
1 teaspoon dried thyme
½ teaspoon red pepper flakes
8 ounces (227 g) cremini mushrooms, trimmed and sliced
1 cup chopped onion
1¾ cups water
1 teaspoon kosher salt
1 teaspoon black pepper
8 ounces (227 g) fettuccine, broken in half
8 ounces (227 g) Mascarpone cheese
1 cup shredded Parmesan cheese
2 teaspoons fresh thyme leaves, for garnish

1. Press the Sauté button on the Instant Pot and melt the butter. Add the garlic, thyme, and red pepper flakes to the pot and sauté for 30 seconds. Stir in the mushrooms, onion, water, salt and pepper.
2. Add the fettuccine, pushing it down into the liquid. Add the Mascarpone on top of the pasta. Do not stir.
3. Lock the lid. Select the Manual mode and set the cooking time for 5 minutes on High Pressure. Once the timer goes off, perform a natural pressure release for 5 minutes, then release any remaining pressure. Carefully open the lid.
4. Stir in the Parmesan cheese.
5. Divide the pasta among four dishes, garnish with the thyme and serve.

Mexican Rice

Prep time: 5 minutes | Cook time: 14 to 16 minutes | Serves 4 to 6

1 tablespoon olive oil
¼ cup diced onion
2 cups long grain white rice
1 cup salsa
2⅓ cups chicken stock
1 teaspoon salt

1. Press the Sauté button on the Instant Pot and heat the olive oil.
2. Add the diced onion and sauté for 2 to 3 minutes until translucent.
3. Add the white rice and cook for an additional 2 to 3 minutes. Stir in the remaining ingredients.
4. Lock the lid. Select the Manual mode and set the cooking time for 10 minutes at High Pressure.
5. Once cooking is complete, do a natural pressure release for 10 minutes, then release any remaining pressure. Carefully open the lid.
6. Fluff the rice with the rice spatula or fork. Serve warm.

Simple Wild Brown Rice

Prep time: 2 mins, Cook Time: 20 mins, Servings: 6 to 8

- 2 tbsps. olive oil
- 3¾ cups water
- 3 cups wild brown rice
- Salt, to taste

1. Combine the oil, water, and brown rice in the pot.
2. Season with salt.
3. Lock the lid. Select the Multigrain mode, then set the timer for 20 minutes on Low Pressure.
4. Once the timer goes off, do a natural pressure release for 5 minutes. Carefully open the lid.
5. Fluff the rice with a fork.
6. Serve immediately.

Mustard Macaroni and Cheese

Prep time: 10 minutes | Cook time: 6 minutes | Serves 4 to 6

1 pound (454 g) elbow macaroni

4 cups chicken broth or vegetable broth, low sodium

3 tablespoons unsalted butter

½ cup sour cream

3 cups shredded Cheddar cheese, about 12 ounces (340 g)

½ cup shredded Parmesan cheese, about 2 ounces (57 g)

1½ teaspoons yellow mustard

⅛ teaspoon cayenne pepper

1. Add the macaroni, broth, and butter to your Instant Pot.
2. Secure the lid. Press the Manual button on the Instant Pot and set the cooking time for 6 minutes on High Pressure.
3. Once cooking is complete, perform a quick pressure release. Carefully remove the lid.
4. Stir in the sour cream, cheese, mustard, and cayenne pepper.
5. Let stand for 5 minutes. Stir well.
6. Serve immediately.

Spinach and Mushroom Pasta

Prep time: 5 minutes | Cook time: 10 minutes | Serves 4

1 tablespoon oil

8 ounces (227 g) mushrooms, minced

½ teaspoon kosher salt

½ teaspoon black ground pepper

8 ounces (227 g) uncooked spaghetti pasta

1¾ cups water

5 ounces (142 g) spinach

½ cup pesto

⅓ cup grated Parmesan cheese

1. Press the Sauté button on the Instant Pot and heat the oil. Add the mushrooms, salt and pepper to the pot and sauté for 5 minutes. Add the pasta and water.
2. Set the lid in place. Select the Manual mode and set the cooking time for 5 minutes on High Pressure. When the timer goes off, do a quick pressure release. Carefully open the lid.

3. Stir in the spinach, pesto, and cheese. Serve immediately.

Feta and Arugula Pasta Salad

Prep time: 10 minutes | Cook time: 8 minutes | Serves 4 to 6

1 pound (454 g) dry rotini pasta

Water as needed, to cover the pasta

2 cups arugula or spinach, chopped

1 cup feta cheese, diced

2 Roma or plum tomatoes, diced

2 garlic cloves, minced

1 red bell pepper, diced

2 tablespoons white wine vinegar

⅓ cup extra-virgin olive oil

Salt and ground black pepper, to taste

1. Place the pasta and water in your Instant Pot.
2. Secure the lid. Press the Manual button on your Instant Pot and set the cooking time for 8 minutes on High Pressure.
3. Once the timer goes off, do a quick pressure release. Carefully open the lid.
4. Drain the pasta and set aside.
5. Mix together the arugula, feta, tomatoes, garlic, bell pepper, vinegar, and olive oil in a large bowl.
6. Fold in the pasta. Sprinkle with salt and pepper. Stir well.
7. Serve immediately.

Caper and Olive Pasta

Prep time: 10 minutes | Cook time: 5 minutes | Serves 4

3 cloves garlic, minced

4 cups of pasta such as penne or fusilli (short pasta)

4 cups of pasta sauce (homemade or store-bought)

3 cups of water, plus more as needed

1 tablespoon of capers

½ cup of Kalamata olives, sliced

¼ teaspoon. of crushed red pepper flakes

Salt and pepper, to taste

1. Press the Sauté button on your Instant Pot and add the garlic.

2. Add a splash of water and cook for about 30 seconds until fragrant.

3. Mix in the pasta, pasta sauce, water, capers, olives, and crushed red pepper flakes and stir to combine.

4. Lock the lid. Press the Manual button on the Instant Pot and set the cooking time for 5 minutes on High Pressure.

5. Once the timer goes off, use a quick pressure release. Carefully remove the lid.

6. Fold in the pasta and sprinkle with salt and pepper. Stir well.

7. Serve immediately.

Penne Pasta with Tomato-Vodka Sauce

Prep time: 5 minutes | Cook time: 4 minutes | Serves 2

½ cup uncooked penne pasta

½ cup crushed tomatoes

1 cup water

⅛ cup coconut oil

1 tablespoon vodka

1 teaspoon garlic powder

½ teaspoon salt

¼ teaspoon paprika

½ cup coconut cream

⅛ cup minced cilantro

1. Add all the ingredients, except for the coconut cream and cilantro, to the Instant Pot and stir to combine.

2. Set the lid in place. Select the Manual mode and set the cooking time for 4 minutes on High Pressure. When the timer goes off, do a quick pressure release. Carefully open the lid.

3. Stir in the coconut cream and fresh cilantro and serve hot.

Zucchini Penne Pasta

Prep time: 10 minutes | Cook time: 10 minutes | Serves 5

1 tablespoon butter

1 yellow onion, thinly sliced

1 shallot, finely chopped

Salt and black pepper, to taste

2 garlic cloves, minced

12 mushrooms, thinly sliced

1 zucchini, thinly sliced

Pinch of dried oregano

Pinch of dried basil

2 cups water

1 cup vegetable stock

2 tablespoons soy sauce

Splash of sherry wine

15 ounces (425 g) penne pasta

5 ounces (142 g) tomato paste

1. Press the Sauté button on the Instant Pot and melt the butter. Add the onion, shallot, salt and pepper to the pot and sauté for 3 minutes. Add the garlic and continue to sauté for 1 minute.

2. Stir in the mushrooms, zucchini, oregano and basil. Cook for 1 minute more. Pour in the water, stock, soy sauce and wine. Add the penne, tomato paste, salt and pepper.

3. Set the lid in place. Select the Manual mode and set the cooking time for 5 minutes on High Pressure. When the timer goes off, do a quick pressure release. Carefully open the lid.

4. Serve hot.

Cherry Tomato Farfalle with Pesto

Prep time: 5 minutes | Cook time: 8 to 9 minutes | Serves 2 to 4

1½ cup farfalle

4 cups water

¾ cup vegan pesto sauce

1 cup cherry tomatoes, quartered

1. Place the farfalle and water in your Instant Pot.

2. Secure the lid. Press the Manual button and cook for 7 minutes at High Pressure.

3. Once cooking is complete, do a quick pressure release. Carefully remove the lid.

4. Drain the pasta and transfer it back to the pot.

5. Stir in the sauce.

6. Press the Sauté button on your Instant Pot and cook for 1 to 2 minutes.

7. Fold in the tomatoes and stir to combine.

8. Transfer to a serving dish and serve immediately.

Tuna Noodle Casserole with Cheese

Prep time: 10 minutes | Cook time: 3 minutes | Serves 6

12 ounces (340 g) egg noodles

1 (8- to 12-ounce / 227- to 340-g) can tuna albacore chunk preferred, drained

1 cup of frozen peas

1 cup of mushrooms, sliced

3 cup of chicken broth

1 teaspoon of salt

1 teaspoon of garlic powder

½ teaspoon of pepper (optional)

1.5 cup of cheese

1 cup half and half

Hot water and cornstarch as needed

1. Stir together all the ingredients except the cheese and half and half in your Instant Pot.
2. Lock the lid. Press the Manual button and cook for 3 minutes at High Pressure.
3. Once cooking is complete, use a quick pressure release. Carefully remove the lid.
4. Add the cheese and half and half and stir until the cheese has melted. Let stand for about 5 minutes until thickened.
5. Combine some hot water and some cornstarch in a medium bowl and add to the pot to thicken quicker.
6. Serve.

Vegan Rice Pudding

Prep time: 6 mins, Cook Time: 18 mins, Servings: 6

- ⅔ cup Jasmine rice, rinsed and drained
- ¼ cup granulated sugar
- 3 cups almond milk
- Salt, to taste
- 1½ tsps. vanilla extract

1. Add all the ingredients, except vanilla extract, to the Instant Pot.
2. Lock the lid. Select the Manual mode, then set the timer for 18 minutes at Low Pressure.
3. Once the timer goes off, do a natural pressure release for 10 minutes, then release any remaining pressure. Carefully open the lid.

4. Stir in the vanilla extract and cool for 10 minutes, then serve.

Vegetable Basmati Rice

Prep time: 10 minutes | Cook time: 9 to 10 minutes | Serves 6 to 8

3 tablespoons olive oil

3 cloves garlic, minced

1 large onion, finely chopped

3 tablespoons chopped cilantro stalks

1 cup garden peas, frozen

1 cup sweet corn, frozen

2 cups basmati rice, rinsed

1 teaspoon turmeric powder

¼ teaspoon salt

3 cups chicken stock

2 tablespoons butter (optional)

1. Press the Sauté button on the Instant Pot and heat the olive oil.
2. Add the garlic, onion, and cilantro and sauté for 5 to 6 minutes, stirring occasionally, or until the garlic is fragrant.
3. Stir in the peas, sweet corn, and rice. Scatter with the turmeric and salt. Pour in the chicken stock and stir to combine.
4. Lock the lid. Select the Manual mode and set the cooking time for 4 minutes at High Pressure.
5. Once cooking is complete, do a quick pressure release. Carefully open the lid.
6. You can add the butter, if desired. Serve warm.

Vegetable Pasta

Prep time: 10 minutes | Cook time: 7 minutes | Serves 4 to 6

2 cups dried pasta

1 cup water

½ jar spaghetti sauce

½ can chickpeas, rinsed and drained

½ can black olives, rinsed and drained

½ cup frozen spinach

½ cup frozen lima beans

½ squash, shredded

½ zucchini, sliced

½ tablespoon Italian seasoning

½ teaspoon cumin

½ teaspoon garlic powder

1. Add all the ingredients to the Instant Pot and stir to combine.

2. Press the Manual button on the Instant Pot and set the cooking time for 7 minutes on High Pressure.

3. Once cooking is complete, perform a natural pressure release for 10 minutes and then release any remaining pressure. Carefully open the lid.

4. Transfer to a serving dish and serve immediately.

Vegetarian Thai Pineapple Fried Rice

Prep time: 10 minutes | Cook time: 10 minutes | Serves 4

1 tablespoon corn oil

3 tablespoons cashews

¼ cup finely chopped onion

¼ cup finely chopped scallions, white parts only

2 green Thai chiles, finely chopped

1 cup canned pineapple chunks

2 tablespoons roughly chopped fresh basil leaves

½ teaspoon curry powder

¼ teaspoon ground turmeric

2 teaspoons soy sauce

1 teaspoon kosher salt

1 cup steamed short-grain white rice

1¼ cups water

1. Press the Sauté button on the Instant Pot and heat the oil.

2. Once hot, add the cashews and stir for 1 minute. Add the onion, scallions, and chiles, and sauté for 3 to 4 minutes, until the onion is translucent.

3. Mix in the pineapple, basil, curry powder, turmeric, soy sauce, and salt. Add the rice and water and stir to combine.

4. Secure the lid. Select the Manual mode and set the cooking time for 3 minutes at High Pressure.

5. Once cooking is complete, do a natural pressure release for 3 minutes, then release any remaining pressure. Carefully open the lid.

6. Let the rice rest for 15 minutes. Remove the bay leaves. Using a fork, fluff the rice and serve hot.

Vinegary Brown Rice Noodles

Prep time: 5 minutes | Cook time: 3 minutes | Serves 6

8 ounces (227 g) uncooked brown rice noodles

2 cups water

½ cup soy sauce

2 tablespoons brown sugar

2 tablespoons white vinegar

2 tablespoons butter

1 tablespoon chili garlic paste

2 red bell peppers, thinly sliced

Topping:

Green onions

Peanuts

Sesame seeds

1. Add all the ingredients, except for the red bell peppers, to the Instant Pot and stir to combine.

2. Set the lid in place. Select the Manual mode and set the cooking time for 3 minutes on High Pressure. When the timer goes off, do a quick pressure release. Carefully open the lid.

3. Stir in the red bell peppers. Sprinkle with the green onions, peanuts and sesame seeds. Serve immediately.

Wild Rice and Basmati Pilaf

Prep time: 5 minutes | Cook time: 35 minutes | Serves 6

2 tablespoon olive oil

2 brown onions, minced

2 cloves garlic, minced

12 ounces (340 g) mushrooms, sliced

½ teaspoon salt

6 sprigs fresh thyme

2 cups broth

2 cups wild rice and basmati rice mixture

½ cup pine nuts

½ cup minced parsley

1. Set your Instant Pot to Sauté. Add the olive oil and onions and cook for 6 minutes.

2. Add minced garlic and cook for 1 minute more. Place the remaining ingredients, except for nuts and parsley, into the Instant Pot and stir well.

3. Lock the lid. Select the Manual mode and set the cooking time for 28 minutes at High Pressure.

4. When the timer beeps, perform a natural pressure release for 15 minutes, then release any remaining pressure. Carefully remove the lid.

5. Sprinkle with the pine nuts and parsley, then serve.

CHAPTER 10 GRAINS AND BEANS

Curried Sorghum with Golden Raisins

Prep time: 10 minutes | Cook time: 20 minutes | Serves 4

1 cup sorghum
3 cups water
Salt, to taste
1 cup milk
2 teaspoons sugar
3 tablespoons rice wine vinegar
1 tablespoon curry powder
½ teaspoon chili powder
2 cups carrots
¼ cup finely chopped green onion
½ cup golden raisins

1. Combine the sorghum, water, and salt in the Instant Pot.
2. Secure the lid. Select the Manual mode and set the cooking time for 20 minutes at High Pressure.
3. Once cooking is complete, do a quick pressure release. Carefully open the lid.
4. In a medium bowl, add the milk, sugar, vinegar, salt, curry powder, and chili powder and whisk well.
5. Drain the sorghum and transfer to a large bowl. Add the milk mixture, carrots, green onion, and raisins. Stir to combine and serve.

Simple Instant Pot Pearl Barley

Prep time: 2 minutes | Cook time: 25 minutes | Serves 4

3 cups water
1½ cups pearl barley, rinsed
Salt, to taste
Peanut butter, to taste (optional)

1. Combine the water, barley, and salt in the Instant Pot.
2. Lock the lid. Select the Manual mode and set the cooking time for 25 minutes at High Pressure.
3. Once cooking is complete, do a natural pressure release for 15 minutes, then release any remaining pressure. Carefully open the lid.
4. Add the peanut butter to taste, if desired. Serve hot.

Vegetable Biryani

Prep time: 10 minutes | Cook time: 15 minutes | Serves 6

2 tablespoons butter
3 cardamom seeds
3 whole cloves
2 dried bay leaves
1 (2-inch) cinnamon stick
1 onion, finely chopped
2 garlic cloves, finely chopped
2 teaspoons finely chopped fresh ginger
1½ cups roughly chopped fresh mint leaves
2 tomatoes, finely chopped
1½ teaspoons kosher salt
2 teaspoons ground coriander
1 teaspoon red chili powder
2 tablespoons plain Greek yogurt, plus more for serving
2 cups mixed vegetables
4 tablespoons finely chopped fresh cilantro, divided
1½ cups basmati rice
2¼ cups water

1. Set your Instant Pot to Sauté and melt the butter.
2. Add the cardamom, cloves, bay leaves, and cinnamon stick. Stir-fry for 30 seconds, then add the onion, garlic, ginger, and mint leaves. Sauté for 3 to 4 minutes until the onion is translucent.
3. Stir in the tomatoes and salt. Loosely place the lid on top and cook for 3 minutes, or until the tomatoes are softened.
4. Add the coriander, chili powder, and yogurt. Mix well and cook for 2 minutes more. Add the mixed vegetables and 2 tablespoons of cilantro, and mix well. Stir in the rice and water.
5. Secure the lid. Select the Manual mode and set the cooking time for 4 minutes at High Pressure.
6. Once cooking is complete, do a natural pressure release for 3 minutes, then release any remaining pressure. Carefully open the lid.
7. Let the rice cool for 15 minutes and remove the bay leaves. Using a fork, fluff the rice and stir in the remaining 2 tablespoons of cilantro. Serve hot with additional yogurt.

Pepper and Egg Oatmeal Bowl

Prep time: 5 minutes | Cook time: 6 to 7 minutes | Serves 2

1½ cups vegetable broth

½ cup steel-cut oats

1 tomato, puréed

Kosher salt and freshly ground black pepper, to taste

2 teaspoons olive oil

1 onion, chopped

2 bell peppers, deseeded and sliced

2 eggs, beaten

1. Add the vegetable broth, oats, tomato, salt and black pepper to the Instant Pot and stir to combine.
2. Set the lid in place. Select the Manual setting and set the cooking time for 3 minutes on High Pressure. When the timer goes off, perform a natural pressure release for 20 minutes, then release any remaining pressure. Open the lid. Transfer the oatmeal to bowls.
3. Heat the olive oil in a skillet over medium-high heat. Add the onion and peppers to the skillet and sauté for 3 to 4 minutes, or until tender. Add the beaten eggs and continue to cook until they are set.
4. Spread the egg mixture over the oatmeal and serve warm.

Farro and Cherry Salad

Prep time: 5 minutes | Cook time: 40 minutes | Serves 4 to 6

3 cups water

1 cup whole grain farro, rinsed

1 tablespoon extra-virgin olive oil

1 tablespoon apple cider vinegar

2 cups cherries, cut into halves

¼ cup chopped green onions

1 teaspoon lemon juice

Salt, to taste

10 mint leaves, chopped

1. Combine the water and farro in the Instant Pot.
2. Lock the lid. Select the Manual mode and set the cooking time for 40 minutes at High Pressure.
3. When the timer beeps, perform a quick pressure release. Carefully remove the lid.

4. Drain the farro and transfer to a bowl. Stir in the olive oil, vinegar, cherries, green onions, lemon juice, salt, and mint. Serve immediately.

Greek Quinoa Bowl

Prep time: 10 minutes | Cook time: 13 minutes | Serves 4

1 tablespoon olive oil

3 cloves garlic, minced

1 cup chopped red onion

½ cup quinoa

2 cups chopped tomatoes

2 cups spinach, torn

2 cups chopped zucchini

2 cups vegetable broth

½ cup chopped black olives

½ cup pine nuts

1. Set your Instant Pot to Sauté and heat the olive oil.
2. Add the garlic and onion and sauté for approximately 5 minutes, stirring frequently.
3. Add the remaining ingredients, except for the pine nuts, to the Instant Pot and stir to combine.
4. Secure the lid. Select the Manual mode and set the cooking time for 8 minutes at High Pressure.
5. Once cooking is complete, do a natural pressure release for 10 minutes, then release any remaining pressure. Carefully open the lid.
6. Fluff the quinoa and stir in the pine nuts, then serve.

Beetroot with Green Beans

Prep time: 15 minutes | Cook time: 5 minutes | Serves 2 to 3

1 cup water

1 cup green beans, cut into ½-inch pieces

1 large beetroot, diced small, around ½-inch pieces

1½ tablespoons olive oil

½ teaspoon mustard seeds

2 teaspoons split and dehusked black gram lentils

2 teaspoons chickpeas

2 dried red chilies, broken

⅛ teaspoon asafetida

12 curry leaves

⅛ teaspoon turmeric powder

½ teaspoon salt

⅓ cup fresh grated coconut

1. Pour the water in the Instant Pot. Put the chopped green beans and beetroot in a steamer basket and then put the steamer basket in the pot.

2. Close the lid. Press the Steam button and set the time to 2 minutes on High Pressure.

3. When timer beeps, do a quick pressure release. Open the lid. Remove the steamer basket from the pot and transfer the steamed vegetables to a bowl. Set aside.

4. Press the Sauté button, add the oil and mustard seeds. Heat for a few seconds until pop.

5. Add the lentils and chickpeas and cook for 2 minutes, or until golden.

6. Add the dried red chilies and asafetida and sauté for a few seconds.

7. Add the curry leaves, stir, then add the steamed vegetables, turmeric powder and salt.

8. Toss to combine well, then fold in the fresh grated coconut. Transfer to a serving dish and serve.

Asparagus and Green Pea Risotto

Prep time: 10 minutes | Cook time: 10 minutes | Serves 4

1½ cups Arborio rice

4 cups water, divided

1 tablespoon vegetable bouillon

1 cup fresh sweet green peas

1½ cups chopped asparagus

2 tablespoons nutritional yeast

1 tablespoon lemon juice

Fresh chopped thyme, for garnish

Salt and ground black pepper, to taste

1. Add the rice, 3½ cups of water, and vegetable bouillon to the Instant Pot. Put the lid on.

2. Select Manual setting and set a timer for 5 minutes on High Pressure.

3. When timer beeps, perform a natural pressure release for 5 minutes, then release any remaining pressure. Open the lid.

4. Stir in the peas, asparagus, nutritional yeast, remaining water, and lemon juice.

5. Set to Sauté function. Sauté for 5 minutes or until the asparagus and peas are soft.

6. Spread the thyme on top and sprinkle with salt and pepper before serving.

Black Bean and Quinoa Bowl with Beef

Prep time: 10 minutes | Cook time: 14 to 15 minutes | Serves 4

1 tablespoon olive oil

1 pound (454 g) ground beef

Salt and black pepper, to taste

1 cup fresh corn

1 onion, finely diced

1 red bell pepper, chopped

1 jalapeño pepper, minced

2 garlic cloves, minced

1 teaspoon ground cumin

1 tablespoon chili seasoning

1 (14-ounce / 397-g) can diced tomatoes

1 (8-ounce / 227-g) can black beans, rinsed

2½ cups chicken broth

1 cup quick-cooking quinoa

1 cup grated Cheddar cheese

2 tablespoons chopped cilantro

2 limes, cut into wedges for garnish

1. Press the Sauté button on the Instant Pot and heat the olive oil. Add the beef to the pot and sauté for 5 minutes, or until lightly browned. Season with salt and pepper.

2. Stir in the corn, onion, red bell pepper, jalapeño pepper and garlic. Cook for 5 minutes, or until the bell pepper is tender. Season with the cumin and chili seasoning. Stir in the tomatoes, black beans, chicken broth and quinoa.

3. Lock the lid. Select the Manual setting and set the cooking time for 1 minute at High Pressure. Once the timer goes off, use a quick pressure release. Carefully open the lid.

4. Select the Sauté mode. Sprinkle the food with the Cheddar cheese and 1 tablespoon of the cilantro. Cook for 3 to 4 minutes, or until cheese melts.

5. Spoon quinoa into serving bowls and garnish with the remaining 1 tablespoon of the cilantro and lime wedges. Serve warm.

Lentils with Spinach

Prep time: 15 minutes | Cook time: 15 minutes | Serves 2

1 tablespoon olive oil
½ teaspoon cumin seeds
¼ teaspoon mustard seeds
3 cloves garlic, finely chopped
1 green chili, finely chopped
1 large tomato, chopped
1½ cups spinach, finely chopped
¼ teaspoon turmeric powder
½ teaspoon salt
¼ cup split pigeon peas, rinsed
¼ cup split red lentil, rinsed
1½ cups water
¼ teaspoon garam masala
2 teaspoons lemon juice
Cilantro, for garnish

1. Press the Sauté button on the Instant Pot. Add the oil and then the cumin seeds and mustard seeds.
2. Let the seeds sizzle for a few seconds and then add the garlic and green chili. Sauté for 1 minute or until fragrant.
3. Add the tomato and cook for 1 minute. Add the chopped spinach, turmeric powder and salt, and cook for 2 minutes.
4. Add the rinsed peas and lentils and stir. Pour in the water and put the lid on.
5. Press the Manual button and set the cooking time for 10 minutes on High Pressure.
6. When timer beeps, let the pressure release naturally for 5 minutes, then release any remaining pressure.
7. Open the pot and add the garam masala, lemon juice and cilantro. Serve immediately.

Mediterranean Couscous Salad

Prep time: 20 minutes | Cook time: 2 minutes | Serves 6

Couscous:
1 cup couscous
2¾ cups water, divided
Salad:
½ cup salad greens (such as a mix of spinach, arugula, and red and green lettuce leaves)
4 tablespoons finely chopped carrot
4 tablespoons finely chopped black olives
4 tablespoons finely chopped cucumber
½ cup thinly sliced red onion, marinated in 2 tablespoons each of lemon juice and water for 20 minutes, then drained
½ cup shredded red cabbage, marinated in 2 tablespoons each of lemon juice and water for 20 minutes, then drained
1 teaspoon kosher salt
1 teaspoon freshly ground black pepper
2 tablespoons extra-virgin olive oil

1. Combine the couscous and 1¼ of cups water in a heatproof bowl.
2. Pour the remaining 1½ cups of water into the Instant Pot and insert a trivet. Place the bowl on the trivet.
3. Secure the lid. Select the Manual mode and set the cooking time for 2 minutes at High Pressure.
4. Once cooking is complete, do a natural pressure release for 5 minutes, then release any remaining pressure. Carefully open the lid.
5. Let the couscous cool for 15 minutes before fluffing with a fork.
6. Assemble the salad: Add the salad greens, carrot, olives, cucumber, onion, cabbage, salt, pepper, and olive oil to the couscous. Mix gently and serve immediately.

Moong Bean with Cabbage

Prep time: 10 minutes | Cook time: 8 minutes | Serves 2

2 teaspoons olive oil
½ teaspoon mustard seeds
1 small red onion, chopped
2 green chilies, sliced
5 cups cabbage, shredded
½ cup split moong bean, rinsed
½ teaspoon turmeric powder
½ teaspoon salt
⅓ cup water
¼ cup fresh dill, chopped
Garam masala, for topping

1. Press the Sauté button on the Instant Pot. Add the oil and the mustard seeds. Heat for a few seconds until the mustard seeds pop.
2. Add the onion and sliced green chilies. Sauté for 2 minutes or until softened.
3. Add the shredded cabbage and sauté for 1 minute.
4. Add the moong bean, turmeric powder, and salt and mix well.
5. Pour in the water and close the pot. Press the Manual button and set the timer for 5 minutes on High Pressure.
6. When timer beeps, let the pressure release naturally for 5 minutes, then release any remaining pressure.
7. Open the pot, add the chopped dill, and sprinkle with garam masala. Stir to mix well. Serve hot.

Mujadara (Lebanese Lentils and Rice)

Prep time: 5 minutes | Cook time: 15 minutes | Serves 6
⅓ cup dried brown lentils
2 tablespoons vegetable oil
1 large yellow onion, sliced
1 teaspoon kosher salt, or more to taste
1 cup basmati rice, rinsed and drained
½ teaspoon ground cumin
½ teaspoon ground coriander
2 cups water

1. Place the lentils in a small bowl. Cover with hot water and soak for 15 to 20 minutes, then drain.
2. Press the Sauté button on the Instant Pot and heat the oil.
3. Add the onion and season with a little salt and cook, stirring, until the onions begin to crisp around the edges but are not burned, 5 to 10 minutes. Remove half the onions from the pot and reserve as a garnish.
4. Add the soaked lentils, rice, cumin, coriander, salt, and water, stirring well.
5. Lock the lid. Select the Manual mode and set the cooking time for 6 minutes at High Pressure.
6. When the timer beeps, perform a natural pressure release for 10 minutes, then release any remaining pressure. Carefully remove the lid.
7. Transfer to a serving dish. Sprinkle with the reserved cooked onions and serve.

Mushroom Barley Risotto

Prep time: 10 minutes | Cook time: 40 minutes | Serves 6
3 tablespoons butter
1 onion, finely chopped
1 cup coarsely chopped shiitake mushrooms
1 cup coarsely chopped cremini mushrooms
1 cup coarsely chopped brown bella mushrooms
1 teaspoon kosher salt
1 teaspoon freshly ground black pepper
1 teaspoon Italian dried herb seasoning
1 cup pearl barley
1 (32-ounce / 907-g) container vegetable broth
½ cup shredded Parmesan cheese

1. Set your Instant Pot to Sauté and melt the butter.
2. Add the onion and cook for about 3 minutes, or until the onion is translucent. Mix in the mushrooms, salt, pepper, and Italian seasoning. Cook for 5 to 6 minutes or until the mushrooms shrink. Stir in the barley and broth.
3. Secure the lid. Select the Manual mode and set the cooking time for 30 minutes at High Pressure.
4. Once cooking is complete, do a natural pressure release for 10 minutes, then release any remaining pressure. Carefully open the lid.
5. Stir in the Parmesan cheese. Serve hot.

Farro Risotto with Mushroom

Prep time: 10 minutes | Cook time: 30 minutes | Serves 3
½ cup farro
2 tablespoons barley
3 cups chopped mushrooms
1 tablespoon red curry paste
1 jalapeño pepper, seeded and chopped
1 tablespoon shallot powder
2 tablespoons onion powder
Salt and pepper, to taste
4 garlic cloves, minced
1½ cups water
2 tomatoes, diced
Chopped cilantro, for serving

Chopped scallions, for serving

1. Combine all the ingredients, except for the tomatoes, cilantro, and scallion, in the Instant Pot.
2. Secure the lid. Select the Manual mode and set the cooking time for 30 minutes at High Pressure.
3. Once cooking is complete, do a quick pressure release. Carefully open the lid.
4. Stir in the tomatoes and let sit for 2 to 3 minutes until warmed through. Sprinkle with the cilantro and scallions and serve.

Black-Eyed Pea Rice Bowl

Prep time: 15 minutes | Cook time: 14 minutes | Serves 4

1 teaspoon extra-virgin olive oil
1 large onion, diced
2 carrots, diced
3 celery stalks, diced
3 cloves garlic, minced
1 cup dried black-eyed peas
½ cup white rice
1 medium tomato, diced
1 teaspoon dried oregano
1 teaspoon dried parsley
¼ teaspoon ground cumin
1 teaspoon crushed red pepper
¼ teaspoon ground black pepper
¼ cup tomato paste
2½ cups vegetable broth
2 tablespoons lemon juice
Salt, to taste

1. Select the Sauté setting of the Instant Pot and heat the oil until shimmering.
2. Add the onion, carrots, celery and garlic and sauté for 6 minutes or until tender.
3. Add the black-eyed peas, rice, tomato, oregano, parsley, cumin red and black peppers, tomato paste and broth to the onion mixture and stir to combine.
4. Put the lid on. Select the Manual setting and set the timer for 8 minutes at High Pressure.
5. When timer beeps, let the pressure release naturally for 5 minutes, then release any remaining pressure. Open the lid.

6. Mix in the lemon juice and salt before serving.

Spinach and Tomato Couscous

Prep time: 10 minutes | Cook time: 8 minutes | Serves 4

2 tablespoons butter
1 cup couscous
1¼ cups water
½ cup chopped spinach
1½ tomatoes, chopped

1. Set your Instant Pot to Sauté and melt the butter.
2. Add the couscous and cook for 1 minute.
3. Pour in the water and stir well.
4. Lock the lid. Select the Manual mode and set the cooking time for 5 minutes at High Pressure.
5. When the timer beeps, perform a quick pressure release. Carefully remove the lid.
6. Transfer the couscous to a large bowl. Add the spinach and tomatoes, stir, and serve.

Sumptuous Navy Beans

Prep time: 20 minutes | Cook time: 50 minutes | Serves 10

2 tablespoons extra-virgin olive oil
1 green bell pepper, deseeded and chopped
1 onion, minced
1 jalapeño pepper, minced
3 garlic cloves, minced
6 ounces (170 g) tomato paste
¼ cup molasses
1 teaspoon balsamic vinegar
2 cups vegetable broth
1 tablespoon mustard
¼ teaspoon smoked paprika
¼ cup sugar
¼ teaspoon ground black pepper
1 pound (454 g) navy beans, soaked in water for at least 4 hours, drained
2 cups water
Salt, to taste

1. Add the butter to the Instant Pot and select Sauté setting.

2. Add the bell pepper and onion and cook for 4 minutes or until the onion is translucent.

3. Add the jalapeño and garlic and cook for 1 minute or until fragrant.

4. Meanwhile, combine remaining ingredients in a bowl, except the beans and water, and beat until smooth to make the sauce.

5. Stir the beans, water and sauce mixture in the pot. Secure the lid.

6. Set on Manual mode and set cooking time for 45 minutes on High Pressure.

7. When timer beeps, allow a natural pressure release for 15 minutes, then release any remaining pressure.

8. Remove the lid and stir in the salt before serving.

Super Bean and Grain Burgers

Prep time: 25 minutes | Cook time: 1 hour 15 minutes | Makes 12 patties

1 tablespoon olive oil
½ cup chopped onion
8 cloves garlic, minced
1 cup dried black beans
½ cup quinoa, rinsed
½ cup brown rice
4 cups water
Patties:
½ cup ground flaxseed
1 tablespoon dried marjoram
2 teaspoons smoked paprika
2 teaspoons salt
1 teaspoon ground black pepper
1 teaspoon dried thyme

1. Select the Sauté setting of the Instant Pot and heat the oil until shimmering.

2. Add the onion and sauté for 5 minutes or until transparent.

3. Add the garlic and sauté a minute more or until fragrant.

4. Add the black beans, quinoa, rice and water to the onion mixture and stir to combine.

5. Put the lid on. Set to Manual mode. Set cooking time for 34 minutes on High Pressure.

6. When timer beeps, release the pressure naturally for 15 minutes, then release any remaining pressure. Open the lid.

7. Preheat the oven to 350°F (180°C) and line 2 baking sheets with parchment paper.

8. Mash the beans in the pot, then mix in the ground flaxseed, marjoram, paprika, salt, pepper and thyme.

9. Divide and shape the mixture into 12 patties and put on the baking sheet.

10. Cook in the preheated oven for 35 minutes or until firmed up. Flip the patties halfway through the cooking time.

11. Serve immediately.

Vegetable Fried Millet

Prep time: 10 minutes | Cook time: 25 minutes | Serves 4

1 teaspoon vegetable oil
½ cup thinly sliced oyster mushrooms
1 cup finely chopped leeks
2 garlic cloves, minced
½ cup green lentils, rinsed
1 cup millet, soaked and drained
½ cup sliced bok choy
1 cup chopped asparagus
1 cup chopped snow peas
2¼ cups vegetable stock
Salt and black pepper, to taste
A drizzle of lemon juice
¼ cup mixed chives and parsley, finely chopped

1. Press the Sauté button on the Instant Pot and heat the oil.

2. Cook the mushrooms, leeks, and garlic for 3 minutes. Add lentils and millet, stir, and cook for 4 minutes.

3. Stir in the bok choy, asparagus, snow peas, and vegetable stock.

4. Secure the lid. Select the Manual mode and set the cooking time for 10 minutes at High Pressure.

5. Once cooking is complete, do a quick pressure release. Carefully open the lid.

6. Season to taste with salt and pepper. Serve sprinkled with the lemon juice, chives, and parsley.

White Beans with Poblano and Tomatillos

Prep time: 15 minutes | Cook time: 39 minutes | Serves 6

1 cup chopped poblano, deseeded and stem removed
2 cups chopped tomatillos
1 cup chopped onion
½ jalapeño, deseeded
1½ teaspoons ground cumin
1½ cups dried white beans, soaked for 8 hours, drained
2 teaspoons dried oregano
1½ cups water
Salt and ground black pepper, to taste

1. Add the poblano, tomatillos, onion and jalapeño to a food processor. Pulse to break them into tiny pieces.
2. Set the Sauté setting of the Instant Pot and pour in the blended mixture.
3. Fold in the cumin. Sauté for 4 minutes or until the onion is translucent.
4. Stir in the beans, oregano, and water. Put the lid on.
5. Select the Manual setting and set cooking time for 35 minutes at High Pressure.
6. When timer beeps, allow the pressure to release naturally for 15 minutes, then release any remaining pressure. Open the lid.
7. Sprinkle with salt and pepper before serving.

Za'atar-Spiced Bulgur Wheat Salad

Prep time: 10 minutes | Cook time: 2 minutes | Serves 6

Bulgur Wheat:
1 cup bulgur wheat
2¼ cups water, divided
Salad:
¼ cup finely chopped cucumber
¼ cup finely chopped fresh parsley
2 tablespoons finely chopped fresh mint
2 tablespoons extra-virgin olive oil
2 tablespoons freshly squeezed lemon juice
5 cherry tomatoes, finely chopped
1 teaspoon kosher salt
½ teaspoon freshly ground black pepper
1 teaspoon za'atar spice blend

1. Combine the bulgur wheat and 1¼ cups of water in a heatproof bowl.
2. Pour the remaining 1 cup of water into the Instant Pot and insert a trivet. Place the bowl on the trivet.
3. Secure the lid. Select the Manual mode and set the cooking time for 2 minutes at High Pressure.
4. Once cooking is complete, do a natural pressure release for 5 minutes, then release any remaining pressure. Carefully open the lid.
5. Let the bulgur wheat cool for 20 minutes before fluffing it with a fork.
6. Assemble the salad: Add the cucumber, parsley, mint, olive oil, lemon juice, tomatoes, salt, pepper, and za'atar seasoning to the bulgur wheat. Mix gently and serve immediately.

CHAPTER 11 SOUPS, STEWS, AND CHILIS

Kidney Bean Stew

Prep time: 15 mins, Cook Time: 15 mins, Servings: 2

- 1 cup tomato passata
- 3 tbsps. Italian herbs
- 1lb. cooked kidney beans
- 1 cup low-sodium beef broth

1. Mix all the ingredients in the Instant Pot.
2. Lock the lid. Select the Bean/Chili mode, then set the timer for 15 minutes at High Pressure.
3. Once the timer goes off, do a natural pressure release for 10 minutes, then release any remaining pressure. Carefully open the lid.
4. Serve warm.

Lentil Soup with Garam Masala

Prep time: 5 minutes | Cook time: 15 minutes | Serves 6

1 tablespoon vegetable oil
2 tablespoons finely diced shallot
1 cup diced carrots
1 cup diced celery
½ teaspoon garam masala
½ teaspoon ground cinnamon
½ teaspoon cumin
1 bay leaf
1¾ cups dried brown or green lentils, rinsed and drained
2 cups vegetable broth
3 cups water
¼ to ½ teaspoon sea salt (optional)
Freshly ground black pepper, to taste

1. Set your Instant Pot to Sauté and heat the oil.
2. Add the shallot, carrots, and celery and sauté for 3 to 5 minutes, until the shallot and celery are tender, stirring occasionally.
3. Add the garam masala, cinnamon, cumin, bay leaf, and lentils and stir well. Pour in the vegetable broth and water and stir to mix well.
4. Secure the lid. Select the Manual mode and set the cooking time for 8 minutes at High Pressure.

5. Once cooking is complete, do a natural pressure release for 10 minutes, then release any remaining pressure. Carefully open the lid.
6. Remove the bay leaf and sprinkle with salt (if desired). Season to taste with black pepper and serve.

Tofu and Kale Miso Soup

Prep time: 5 minutes | Cook time: 10 minutes | Serves 6

1 to 2 teaspoons vegetable oil
4 cloves garlic, cut in half
1 small sweet onion, quartered
2 medium carrots, cut into 2- to 3-inch pieces
4 cups low-sodium vegetable broth
1 (12-ounce / 340-g) package silken (light firm) tofu
1 bunch kale (off the stem), plus a few leaves for garnish
¼ cup yellow miso
Ground black pepper, to taste

1. Press the Sauté button on the Instant Pot and heat the oil.
2. Add the garlic, onion, and carrots and sauté for 5 minutes, stirring occasionally.
3. Add the vegetable broth and tofu. Crumble the tofu into pieces with a spoon. Add the kale and stir to incorporate.
4. Secure the lid. Select the Manual mode and set the cooking time for 4 minutes at High Pressure.
5. Once cooking is complete, do a natural pressure release for 10 minutes, then release any remaining pressure. Carefully open the lid.
6. Stir in the miso and blend the soup with an immersion blender until smooth.
7. Season to taste with black pepper and serve garnished with extra kale.

Vegetable Quinoa Stew

Prep time: 10 minutes | Cook time: 15 minutes | Serves 4

2 teaspoons corn oil
1 yellow onion, minced
3 Roma tomatoes, minced
¼ cup frozen corn kernels, thawed to room temperature

1 zucchini, cut into 1-inch chunks

½ cup chopped red bell pepper

1½ cups broccoli florets

¼ cup diced carrot

½ cup quinoa, rinsed

1 teaspoon ground coriander

½ teaspoon paprika

½ teaspoon ground cumin

1 (32-ounce / 907-g) container vegetable broth

2 teaspoons kosher salt

4 tablespoons minced fresh cilantro, divided

1. Press the Sauté button on the Instant Pot and heat the oil. Once hot, add the onion and sauté 5 minutes, stirring occasionally.

2. Add the tomatoes, corn, zucchini, bell pepper, broccoli, and carrot and mix well. Stir in the quinoa, coriander, paprika, cumin, broth, salt, and 2 tablespoons of cilantro.

3. Secure the lid. Select the Manual mode and set the cooking time for 8 minutes at High Pressure.

4. Once cooking is complete, do a natural pressure release for 5 minutes, then release any remaining pressure. Carefully open the lid.

5. Stir in the remaining 2 tablespoons of cilantro and serve hot.

Acorn Squash Chili

Prep time: 15 minutes | Cook time: 16 minutes | Serves 6

1 tablespoon olive oil

½ cup chopped onion

1 cup sliced carrots

1 large celery stalks, chopped

2 cloves garlic, minced

1½ cups cubed acorn squash

10 ounces (283 g) can red kidney beans, drained

10 ounces (283 g) can cannellini beans, drained

2 (10-ounce / 283-g) can crushed tomatoes

¾ cup corn kernels

1 teaspoon Tabasco sauce

1 teaspoon mesquite powder

1 teaspoon chili flakes

1 teaspoon dried oregano

1 teaspoon ground cumin

1 teaspoon smoked paprika

1. Heat the oil in the Instant pot on Sauté mode.

2. Add the onion and carrots. Sauté for 3 minutes or until soft.

3. Add the celery and sauté for 2 minutes. Add the garlic and sauté for 1 minute.

4. Add the remaining ingredients and lock the lid.

5. Select Manual mode and set cooking time for 10 minutes on High Pressure.

6. When timer beeps, use a natural pressure release for 5 minutes, then release any remaining pressure. Open the lid.

7. Serve warm.

Millet and Brown Lentil Chili

Prep time: 10 minutes | Cook time: 20 minutes | Serves 6

2 tablespoons olive oil

1 cup finely diced yellow onion

2 cloves garlic, minced

1 seeded and finely diced fresh jalapeño

½ teaspoon ground cinnamon

1 teaspoon chili powder

1 teaspoon ground cumin

1 cup dried brown lentils, rinsed and drained

1 cup millet, rinsed and drained

½ cup diced summer squash

4 cups diced fresh tomatoes

2 cups bite-size pieces kale

1 bay leaf

2 cups vegetable broth

4 cups water

Juice of 1 lemon

1 tablespoon chopped fresh sweet basil

½ teaspoon sea salt

1. Heat the olive oil in the Instant Pot. Add the onion and cook for 3 to 4 minutes, stirring occasionally, until softened.

2. Add the garlic, stir, then add the jalapeño, cinnamon, chili powder, and cumin and sauté for a few minutes more, until the jalapeño softens.

3. Add the lentils, millet, squash, tomatoes, kale, bay leaf, broth, and water and stir to combine.

4. Cover the lid. Select Manual mode and set cooking time for 8 minutes on High Pressure.

5. When timer beeps, use a natural pressure release for 15 minutes, then release any remaining pressure.

6. Carefully remove the lid. Select Sauté mode and bring to a simmer, then add the lemon juice, basil, and salt.

7. Stir and let simmer for a few minutes more. Serve immediately.

Quinoa and Bean Chili

Prep time: 10 minutes | Cook time: 7 minutes | Serves 6
1 tablespoon olive oil
1 large yellow onion, diced
3 cloves garlic, minced
1 green bell pepper, deseeded and diced
1 cup peeled and diced sweet potato cubes (about 1 inch)
1 (15-ounce / 425-g) can black beans, drained and rinsed
1 (15-ounce / 425-g) can kidney beans, drained and rinsed
½ cup uncooked quinoa, rinsed and drained
1 (4-ounce / 113-g) can diced green chiles
1 (26-ounce / 737-g) box chopped or diced tomatoes
1½ tablespoons chili powder
1 tablespoon ground cumin
½ teaspoon smoked paprika
½ teaspoon sea salt
2 cups vegetable broth
Fresh cilantro leaves, for garnish
1 avocado, sliced, for garnish

1. Select Sauté mode, and heat the oil in the Instant Pot until hot.

2. Add the onion and sauté for 1 minute. Add the garlic, bell pepper, and sweet potatoes, and sauté 1 minute more.

3. Add the black beans, kidney beans, quinoa, chiles, tomatoes, chili powder, cumin, paprika, salt, and broth, and stir.

4. Lock the lid. Select Manual mode and set the cook time for 5 minutes on High Pressure.

5. Once the cook time is complete, quick release the pressure and carefully remove the lid.

6. Serve warm, garnished with cilantro and avocado.

Summer Chili

Prep time: 10 minutes | Cook time: 15 minutes | Serves 6
2 tablespoons olive oil
1 poblano chile or green bell pepper, deseeded and diced
1 jalapeño chile, deseeded and diced
1 celery stalk, diced
2 cloves garlic, minced
1 yellow onion, diced
½ teaspoon fine sea salt, plus more as needed
2 tablespoons chili powder
1 teaspoon dried oregano
½ teaspoon ground cumin
¼ teaspoon cayenne pepper
2 zucchini, diced
1 (15-ounce / 425-g) can peruano beans, rinsed and drained
1 (12-ounce / 340-g) bag frozen corn
1 cup vegetable broth
1 (14.5-ounce / 411-g) can diced fire-roasted tomatoes
¼ cup chopped fresh cilantro
2 green onions, white and tender green parts, thinly sliced

1. Select the Sauté setting on the Instant Pot, add the oil, and heat for 1 minute.

2. Add the poblano and jalapeño chiles, celery, garlic, onion, and salt, and sauté for about 5 minutes, until the vegetables soften.

3. Add the chili powder, oregano, cumin, and cayenne and sauté for about 1 minute more.

4. Add the zucchini, beans, corn, and broth and stir to combine. Pour the tomatoes and their liquid over the top. Do not stir.

5. Secure the lid. Select Manual mode and set the cooking time for 5 minutes at High Pressure.

6. When timer beeps, perform a quick pressure release. Open the pot, give a stir.

7. Ladle the chili into bowls and sprinkle with cilantro and green onions. Serve hot.

Winter Chili

Prep time: 10 minutes | Cook time: 15 minutes | Serves 4 to 6

3 tablespoons olive oil

2 cloves garlic, minced

2 leeks, white and tender green parts, halved lengthwise and thinly sliced

2 jalapeño chiles, deseeded and diced

1 teaspoon fine sea salt

1 canned chipotle chile in adobo sauce, minced

3 tablespoons chili powder

1 cup vegetable broth

2 carrots, peeled and diced

1 (15-ounce / 425-g) can black beans, rinsed and drained

1 (1-pound / 454-g) delicata squash, deseeded and diced

1 (14.5-ounce / 411-g) can diced fire-roasted tomatoes

Chopped fresh cilantro, for serving

1. Select the Sauté setting on the Instant Pot, add the oil and garlic, and heat for 2 minutes, until the garlic is bubbling.
2. Add the leeks, jalapeños, and salt and sauté for 5 minutes, until the leeks are wilted.
3. Add the chipotle chile and chili powder and sauté for 1 minute more. Stir in the broth.
4. Add the carrots, beans and the squash. Pour the tomatoes and their liquid over the top. Do not stir.
5. Secure the lid. Select Manual mode and set the cooking time for 5 minutes at High Pressure.
6. When timer beeps, perform a quick pressure release. Open the pot, give a stir.
7. Ladle the chili into bowls and sprinkle with cilantro. Serve hot.

Salmon Head Soup

Prep time: 6 mins, Cook Time: 12 mins, Servings: 1

- 1 tsp. coconut oil
- 1 onion, sliced
- 3 cups water
- 1 salmon head
- 3-inch ginger piece, slivered
- Salt and pepper, to taste

1. Press the Sauté button on the Instant Pot and heat the coconut oil.
2. Sauté the onion for 3 minutes or until translucent.
3. Pour in the water, then add the salmon head and ginger.
4. Sprinkle salt and pepper for seasoning.
5. Lock the lid. Set on the Manual mode, then set the timer to 10 minutes at Low Pressure.
6. When the timer goes off, perform a quick release.
7. Carefully open the lid. Allow to cool before serving.

Salmon Stew

Prep time: 6 mins, Cook Time:13 mins, Servings: 9

- 2 tbsps. olive oil
- 3 garlic cloves, minced
- 3 cups water
- 3 lbs. salmon fillets
- Salt and pepper, to taste
- 3 cups spinach leaves

1. Press the Sauté button on the Instant Pot and heat the olive oil.
2. Sauté the garlic for a minute until fragrant.
3. Add the water and salmon fillets. Sprinkle salt and pepper for seasoning.
4. Lock the lid. Set on the Manual mode, then set the timer to 10 minutes at Low Pressure.
5. When the timer goes off, perform a quick release.
6. Carefully open the lid. Press the Sauté button and add the spinach.
7. Allow to simmer for 3 minutes.
8. Serve warm.

Broccoli and Brussels Sprout Salad

Prep time: 12 mins, Cook Time: 6 mins, Servings: 6

- 1½ cups water
- 2 tsps. mustard
- 1 head broccoli, cut into florets
- ½ cup walnut oil
- 1 lb. halved Brussels sprouts
- ¼ cup balsamic vinegar

1. Put the water in the Instant Pot and arrange the steamer basket in the pot, then add broccoli and Brussels sprouts.
2. Lock the lid. Select the Manual mode, then set the timer for 4 minutes at High Pressure.
3. Once the timer goes off, do a quick pressure release. Carefully open the lid.
4. Drain the vegetables and transfer to a bowl.
5. Clean the pot and set it to Sauté. Heat the oil and add broccoli and Brussels sprouts. Stir and cook for 1 minute.
6. Drizzle with the vinegar and cook for 1 minute more, then transfer to a bowl.
7. Add the mustard and toss well. Serve immediately or refrigerate to chill.

Beet and Carrot Spread

Prep time: 12 mins, Cook Time: 12 mins, Servings: 6
- 1 bunch basil, chopped
- 8 carrots, chopped
- ¼ cup lemon juice
- 4 beets, peeled and chopped
- 1 cup vegetable stock
1. In the Instant Pot, combine the beets with stock and carrots.
2. Lock the lid. Select the Manual mode and set the cooking time for 12 minutes at High Pressure.
3. Once cooking is complete, do a quick pressure release. Carefully open the lid.
4. Blend the ingredients with an immersion blender, and add the lemon juice and basil, and whisk well. Serve immediately.

Cashew and Hummus Spread

Prep time: 12 mins, Cook Time: 6 mins, Servings: 8
- ¼ cup nutritional yeast
- ¼ tsp. garlic powder
- ½ cup soaked and drained cashews
- 10 oz. hummus
- ½ cup water
1. In the Instant Pot, combine the cashews and water.

2. Lock the lid. Select the Manual mode, then set the timer for 6 minutes at High Pressure.
3. Once the timer goes off, do a quick pressure release. Carefully open the lid.
4. Transfer the cashews to the blender, and add hummus, yeast and garlic powder, and pulse until well combined. Serve immediately.

Cauliflower Tots

Prep time: 15 minutes | Cook time: 23 minutes | Serves 6
1 cup water
1 head cauliflower, broken into florets
2 eggs, beaten
½ cup grated Parmesan cheese
½ cup grated Swiss cheese
2 tablespoons fresh coriander, chopped
1 shallot, chopped
Sea salt and ground black pepper, to taste
1. Add the water to the Instant Pot. Set a steamer basket in the pot.
2. Arrange the cauliflower florets in the steamer basket.
3. Secure the lid. Choose the Manual mode and set the cooking time for 3 minutes at High Pressure.
4. Once cooking is complete, perform a quick pressure release. Carefully open the lid.
5. Mash the cauliflower in a food processor and add the remaining ingredients. Pulse to combine well.
6. Form the mixture into a tater-tot shape with oiled hands.
7. Place cauliflower tots on a lightly greased baking sheet. Bake in the preheated oven at 400ºF (205ºC) for about 20 minutes. Flip halfway through the cooking time.
8. Serve immediately.

Wheat Berry and Celery Salad

Prep time: 15 minutes | Cook time: 40 minutes | Serves 12
1½ tablespoons vegetable oil
6¾ cups water
1½ cups wheat berries
1½ teaspoons Dijon mustard

1 teaspoon granulated sugar

1 teaspoon sea salt

½ teaspoon freshly ground black pepper

¼ cup white wine vinegar

½ cup extra-virgin olive oil

½ small red onion, peeled and diced

2 medium stalks celery, finely diced

1 medium zucchini, peeled, grated and drained

1 medium red bell pepper, deseeded and diced

4 green onions, diced

1⅓ cups frozen corn, thawed

¼ cup diced sun-dried tomatoes

¼ cup chopped fresh Italian flat-leaf parsley

1.   Add the vegetable oil, water, and wheat berries to the Instant Pot.

2.   Set the lid in place. Select the Multigrain mode and set the cooking time for 40 minutes on High Pressure. When the timer goes off, do a quick pressure release. Carefully open the lid.

3.   Fluff the wheat berries with a fork. Drain and transfer to a large bowl.

4.   Make the dressing by processing the mustard, sugar, salt, pepper, vinegar, olive oil, and red onion in a food processor until smooth.

5.   Stir ½ cup of the dressing into the cooled wheat berries. Toss the seasoned wheat berries with the remaining ingredients.

6.   Serve immediately. Cover and refrigerate any leftover dressing up to 3 days.

Broccoli and Cheddar Salad

Prep time: 12 mins, Cook Time: 4 mins, Servings: 4

- 1½ cups water
- 2 tbsps. balsamic vinegar
- 4 oz. cubed Cheddar cheese
- 1 cup mayonnaise
- 1 head broccoli, cut into florets
- ⅛ cup pumpkin seeds

1.   Put the water into the Instant Pot and arrange the steamer basket in the pot, then add the broccoli.

2.   Lock the lid. Select the Manual mode, then set the timer for 3 minutes at High Pressure.

3.   Once the timer goes off, do a quick pressure release. Carefully open the lid.

4.   Drain the broccoli and chop, then transfer to a bowl.

5.   Add the cheese, pumpkin seeds, mayo and vinegar, and toss to combine. Serve immediately.

Shrimp and Tomatoes

Prep time: 12 mins, Cook Time: 4 mins, Servings: 6

- 1 lb. shrimp, shelled and deveined
- 2 tbsps. butter
- 1 cup crumbled feta cheese
- 1½ cups chopped onion
- 15 oz. chopped canned tomatoes

1.   Set the Instant Pot to Sauté and melt the butter.

2.   Add the onion, stir, and cook for 2 minutes.

3.   Add the shrimp and tomatoes and mix well.

4.   Lock the lid. Select the Manual mode, then set the timer for 2 minutes at Low Pressure.

5.   Once the timer goes off, do a quick pressure release. Carefully open the lid.

6.   Divide shrimp and tomatoes mixture into small bowls. Top with feta cheese and serve.

Vegetable Chicken Skewers

Prep time: 15 minutes | Cook time: 5 minutes | Serves 4

1 cup water

1 pound (454 g) chicken breast halves, boneless and skinless

Celery salt and ground black pepper, to taste

½ teaspoon Sriracha sauce

1 zucchini, cut into thick slices

1 cup cherry tomatoes, halved

1 red onion, cut into wedges

¼ cup olives, pitted

1 tablespoon fresh lemon juice

2 tablespoons olive oil

Special Equipment:

4 bamboo skewers

1.   Pour the water in the Instant Pot. Arrange a trivet in the pot. Place the chicken on the trivet.

2.   Secure the lid. Choose Poultry mode and set the cooking time for 5 minutes at High Pressure.

3. Once cooking is complete, perform a natural pressure release for 5 minutes, then release any remaining pressure. Carefully open the lid.

4. Slice the chicken into cubes. Sprinkle chicken cubes with salt, pepper, and drizzle with Sriracha.

5. Thread the chicken cubes, zucchini, cherry tomatoes, onion, and olives onto bamboo skewers. Drizzle the lemon juice and olive oil over and serve.

Barbecue Chicken Meatballs

Prep time: 6 mins, Cook Time: 15 mins, Servings: 8

- 24 oz. frozen chicken meatballs
- ½ tsp. crushed red pepper
- 12 oz. barbecue sauce
- ¼ cup water
- 12 oz. apricot preserves

1. Add all the ingredients to the Instant Pot. Stir to mix well.

2. Lock the lid. Select the Manual mode, then set the timer for 5 minutes at High Pressure.

3. Once the timer goes off, do a quick pressure release. Carefully open the lid.

4. Serve the meatballs on a platter.

Pork and Beef Chili Nachos

Prep time: 25 minutes | Cook time: 45 minutes | Serves 8

1 tablespoon olive oil

1 medium green bell pepper, seeded and diced

1 small red onion, peeled and diced

4 ounces (113 g) ground pork

½ pound (227 g) ground beef

1 (4-ounce / 113-g) can chopped green chiles, with juice

1 (14.5-ounce / 411-g) can diced tomatoes, with juice

1 teaspoon garlic powder

1 tablespoon chili powder

1 teaspoon ground cumin

1 teaspoon salt

4 ounces (113 g) cream cheese

2 Roma tomatoes, deseeded and diced

½ cup shredded Cheddar cheese

4 scallions, sliced

1 bag corn tortilla chips

1. Press the Sauté button on the Instant Pot. Heat the olive oil until shimmering.

2. Add the bell pepper and onion to pot. Sauté for 5 minutes or until onions are translucent. Add the pork and beef and sauté for 5 more minutes.

3. Add the chiles with juice, tomatoes with juice, garlic powder, chili powder, cumin, and salt to pot and stir to combine.

4. Lock the lid. Press the Meat / Stew button and set the time for 35 minutes on High Pressure. When the timer beeps, let pressure release naturally for 10 minutes, then release any remaining pressure.

5. Unlock the lid. Stir in cream cheese until melted and evenly distributed.

6. Transfer chili mixture to a serving dish. Garnish with Roma tomatoes, Cheddar, and scallions. Serve warm with chips.

Chili Endives Platter

Prep time: 12 mins, Cook Time: 7 mins, Servings: 4

- ¼ tsp. chili powder
- 1 tbsp. butter
- 4 trimmed and halved endives
- 1 tbsp. lemon juice
- Salt, to taste

1. Set the Instant Pot to Sauté and melt the butter. Add the endives, salt, chili powder and lemon juice to the pot.

2. Lock the lid. Select the Manual mode, then set the timer for 7 minutes at High Pressure.

3. Once the timer goes off, do a quick pressure release. Carefully open the lid.

4. Divide the endives into bowls. Drizzle some cooking juice over them and serve.

Chinese Flavor Chicken Wings

Prep time: 10 minutes | Cook time: 16 minutes | Serves 6

1 teaspoon Sriracha sauce

2 teaspoons Chinese five-spice powder

¼ cup tamari

¼ cup apple cider vinegar

3 cloves garlic, minced

1 tablespoon light brown sugar

2 tablespoons sesame oil

5 scallions, sliced and separated into whites and greens

3 pounds (1.4 kg) chicken wings, separated at the joint

1 cup water

¼ cup toasted sesame seeds

1. In a large bowl, combine the Sriracha, Chinese five-spice powder, tamari, apple cider vinegar, garlic, brown sugar, sesame oil, and whites of scallions. Stir to mix well. Transfer 2 tablespoons of the sauce mixture to a small bowl and reserve until ready to use.

2. Add wings to the remaining sauce and toss to coat well. Wrap the bowl in plastic and refrigerate for at least 1 hour or up to overnight.

3. Add the water to the Instant Pot and insert a steamer basket. Place the chicken wings in the single layer in the steamer basket. Lock the lid.

4. Press the Manual button and set the cook time for 10 minutes on High Pressure. When the timer beeps, let pressure release naturally for 5 minutes, then release any additional pressure and unlock the lid.

5. Using a slotted spoon, transfer the wings to a baking sheet. Brush with 2 tablespoons of reserved sauce. Broil the wings in the oven for 3 minutes on each side to crisp the chicken.

6. Transfer the wings to a serving dish and garnish with sesame seeds and greens of scallions. Serve immediately.

Citrus Buckwheat and Barley Salad

Prep time: 10 minutes | Cook time: 35 minutes | Serves 4

1 cup wheat berries

1 cup pearl barley

3 cups vegetable broth

¼ cup minced shallots

¼ cup olive oil

¼ cup lemon juice

2 cloves garlic, crushed and minced

¼ cup pine nuts

1 cup finely chopped kale

1 cup chopped tomatoes

½ teaspoon salt

½ teaspoon black pepper

1. In the Instant Pot, combine the wheat berries, pearl barley, vegetable broth and shallots. Mix well.

2. Lock the lid. Select the Manual mode and set the cooking time for 35 minutes on High Pressure. Once the timer goes off, perform a natural pressure release for 20 minutes, then release any remaining pressure. Carefully open the lid.

3. Meanwhile, combine the olive oil, lemon juice and garlic in a bowl. Whisk until well combined.

4. Remove the grains from the cooker and transfer them to a large bowl. Allow them to sit out long enough to cool slightly.

5. Add the dressing, pine nuts, kale and tomatoes to the grains and stir.

6. Season with salt and black pepper, as desired.

7. Serve warm or cover and chill until ready to serve.

Mussel Appetizer

Prep time: 20 minutes | Cook time: 10 minutes | Serves 4

¼ cup olive oil

28 ounces (794 g) canned tomatoes, chopped

2 jalapeño peppers, chopped

½ cup chopped white onion

¼ cup balsamic vinegar

¼ cup veggie stock

2 garlic cloves, minced

2 tablespoons crushed red pepper flakes

2 pounds (907 g) mussels, scrubbed

½ cup chopped basil

Salt, to taste

1. Press the Sauté button on the Instant Pot and heat the olive oil.

2. Add the tomatoes, jalapeño, onion, vinegar, veggie stock, garlic, and red pepper flakes and stir well. Cook for 5 minutes. Stir in the mussels.

3. Secure the lid. Select the Manual mode and set the cooking time for 4 minutes at Low Pressure.

4. Once cooking is complete, do a quick pressure release. Carefully open the lid.

5. Sprinkle with the basil and salt and stir well. Divide the mussels among four bowls and serve.

Jalapeño Peanuts

Prep time: 3 hours 20 minutes | Cook time: 45 minutes | Serves 4

4 ounces (113 g) raw peanuts in the shell

1 jalapeño, sliced

1 tablespoon Creole seasoning

½ tablespoon cayenne pepper

½ tablespoon garlic powder

1 tablespoon salt

1.   Add all ingredients to the Instant Pot. Pour in enough water to cover. Stir to mix well. Use a steamer to gently press down the peanuts.

2.   Secure the lid. Choose the Manual mode and set the cooking time for 45 minutes at High pressure.

3.   Once cooking is complete, perform a natural pressure release for 15 minutes, then release any remaining pressure. Carefully open the lid.

4.   Transfer the peanut and the liquid in a bowl, then refrigerate for 3 hours before serving.

Carrot and Kale Salad

Prep time: 12 mins, Cook Time: 7 mins, Servings: 4

- 1 tbsp. olive oil
- 3 carrots, sliced
- 1 red onion, chopped
- 10 oz. kale, roughly chopped
- ½ cup chicken stock

1.   Set the Instant Pot to Sauté and heat the olive oil.

2.   Add the onion and carrots, stir, and cook for 1 to 2 minutes.

3.   Stir in stock and kale.

4.   Lock the lid. Select the Manual mode, then set the timer for 5 minutes at High Pressure.

5.   Once the timer goes off, do a quick pressure release. Carefully open the lid.

6.   Divide the vegetables among four bowls and serve.

Wild Rice and Kale Salad

Prep time: 12 mins, Cook Time: 25 mins, Servings: 4

- 1 tsp. olive oil
- 1 avocado, peeled, pitted and chopped
- 3 oz. goat cheese, crumbled
- 1 cup cooked wild rice
- 1 bunch kale, roughly chopped

1.   Set the Instant Pot to Sauté and heat the olive oil.

2.   Add the rice and toast for 2 to 3 minutes, stirring often.

3.   Add kale and stir well.

4.   Lock the lid. Select the Manual mode, then set the timer for 20 minutes at Low Pressure.

5.   Once the timer goes off, do a natural pressure release for 10 minutes, then release any remaining pressure. Carefully open the lid.

6.   Add avocado and toss well. Sprinkle the cheese on top and serve.

Endives and Lemon Juice Appetizer

Prep time: 12 mins, Cook Time: 13 mins, Servings: 4

- 3 tbsps. olive oil
- ½ cup chicken stock
- Juice of ½ lemon
- 2 tbsps. chopped parsley
- 8 endives, trimmed

1.   Set the Instant Pot to Sauté and heat the olive oil. Add the endives and cook them for 3 minutes.

2.   Add lemon juice and stock, and whisk well.

3.   Lock the lid. Select the Manual mode, then set the timer for 10 minutes at High Pressure.

4.   Once the timer goes off, do a quick pressure release. Carefully open the lid.

5.   Transfer the endives to a large bowl. Drizzle some cooking juices all over and sprinkle with the chopped parsley before serving.

Potato Cubes

Prep time: 5 minutes | Cook time: 10 minutes | Serves 2

2½ medium potatoes, scrubbed and cubed

1 tablespoon chopped fresh rosemary

½ tablespoon olive oil

Freshly ground black pepper, to taste

1 tablespoon fresh lemon juice

½ cup vegetable broth

1.   Put the potatoes, rosemary, oil, and pepper to the Instant Pot. Stir to mix well.

2. Set to the Sauté mode and sauté for 4 minutes.

3. Fold in the remaining ingredients.

4. Secure the lid and select the Manual function. Set the cooking time for 6 minutes at High Pressure.

5. Once cooking is complete, do a quick release, then open the lid.

6. Serve warm.

Beef Patties with Lentil

Prep time: 25 minutes | Cook time: 25 minutes | Makes 15 patties

1 cup dried yellow lentils

2 cups beef broth

½ pound (227 g) 80/20 ground beef

½ cup chopped old-fashioned oats

2 large eggs, beaten

2 teaspoons Sriracha sauce

2 tablespoons diced yellow onion

½ teaspoon salt

1. Add the lentils and broth to the Instant Pot. Lock the lid.

2. Press the Manual button and set the cook time for 15 minutes on High Pressure. When the timer beeps, let pressure release naturally for 10 minutes, then release any remaining pressure. Unlock the lid.

3. Transfer the lentils to a medium bowl with a slotted spoon. Smash most of the lentils with the back of a spoon until chunky.

4. Add beef, oats, eggs, Sriracha, onion, and salt. Whisk to combine them well. Form the mixture into 15 patties.

5. Cook in a skillet on stovetop over medium-high heat in batches for 10 minutes. Flip the patties halfway through.

6. Transfer patties to serving dish and serve warm.

Little Smokies with Grape Jelly

Prep time: 10 minutes | Cook time: 2 minutes | Serves 4

3 ounces (85 g) little smokies

2 ounces (57 g) grape jelly

¼ teaspoon jalapeño, minced

¼ cup light beer

¼ cup chili sauce

1 tablespoon white vinegar

½ cup roasted vegetable broth

2 tablespoons brown sugar

1. Place all ingredients in the Instant Pot. Stir to mix.

2. Secure the lid. Choose the Manual mode and set the cooking time for 2 minutes at High pressure.

3. Once cooking is complete, perform a quick pressure release. Carefully open the lid.

4. Serve hot.

Steamed Asparagus with Mustard Dip

Prep time: 7 mins, Cook Time: 8 mins, Servings: 4

•   1 tsp. Dijon mustard

•   2 tbsps. mayonnaise

•   Salt and black pepper, to taste

•   1 cup water

•   12 asparagus stems

•   3 tbsps. lemon juice

1. Mix the Dijon mustard, mayonnaise, salt and black pepper in a bowl. Set aside.

2. Set trivet to the Instant Pot and add the water.

3. Place asparagus stems on the trivet and drizzle with lemon juice.

4. Lock the lid. Select the Manual mode, then set the timer for 8 minutes at High Pressure.

5. Once the timer goes off, do a quick pressure release. Carefully open the lid.

6. Dip the asparagus into mustard mixture.

Stuffed Eggs

Prep time: 5 minutes | Cook time: 6 minutes | Serves 4

4 eggs

1½ tablespoons Greek yogurt

1½ tablespoons mayonnaise

½ teaspoon chopped jalapeño

¼ teaspoon onion powder

¼ teaspoon paprika

¼ teaspoon lemon zests

Salt and black pepper, to taste

1 cup water, for the pot

1. Pour the water and insert the trivet in the Instant Pot. Place the eggs on the trivet.

2. Set the lid in place. Select the Manual mode and set the cooking time for 6 minutes on High Pressure. When the timer goes off, do a quick pressure release. Carefully open the lid.

3. Place the eggs into ice-cold water. Peel the eggs, and cut in half, lengthwise. Scoop out the egg yolks and mix them with the remaining ingredients. Fill the hollow eggs with the mixture and serve.

Sweet Roasted Cashews

Prep time: 5 minutes | Cook time: 20 minutes | Serves 2

¾ cup cashews

¼ teaspoon salt

¼ teaspoon ginger powder

1 teaspoon minced orange zest

4 tablespoons honey

1 cup water, for the pot

1. Stir together the honey, orange zest, ginger powder, and salt in a bowl. Add the cashews to the mixture and place it in a ramekin.

2. Pour the water and insert the trivet in the Instant Pot. Place the ramekin on the trivet.

3. Set the lid in place. Select the Manual mode and set the cooking time for 20 minutes on High Pressure. When the timer goes off, do a quick pressure release. Carefully open the lid.

4. Serve immediately.

Three Bean Salad with Parsley

Prep time: 10 minutes | Cook time: 30 minutes | Serves 8

⅓ cup apple cider vinegar

¼ cup granulated sugar

2½ teaspoons salt, divided

½ teaspoon freshly ground black pepper

¼ cup olive oil

½ cup dried chickpeas

½ cup dried kidney beans

1 cup frozen green beans pieces

4 cups water

1 tablespoon vegetable oil

1 cup chopped fresh Italian flat-leaf parsley

½ cup peeled and diced cucumber

½ cup diced red onion

1. For the dressing: In a small bowl, whisk together the vinegar, sugar, 1½ teaspoons of the salt and pepper. While whisking continuously, slowly add the olive oil. Once well combined, cover in plastic and refrigerate.

2. Add the chickpeas, kidney beans, green beans, water, vegetable oil, and the remaining 1 teaspoon of the salt to the Instant Pot. Stir to combine.

3. Lock the lid. Select the Manual mode and set the cooking time for 30 minutes on High Pressure. Once the timer goes off, perform a natural pressure release for 10 minutes, then release any remaining pressure. Carefully open the lid.

4. Transfer the cooked beans to a large mixing bowl. Stir in all the remaining ingredients along with the dressing. Toss to combine thoroughly. Cover and refrigerate for 2 hours before serving.

Thyme Carrots

Prep time: 5 minutes | Cook time: 2 minutes | Serves 2

4 carrots, peeled and cut into sticks

1½ teaspoon fresh thyme

2 tablespoons butter

½ cup water

Salt, to taste

1. Press the Sauté button on the Instant Pot and melt the butter. Add the carrots, thyme, salt, and water to the pot.

2. Set the lid in place. Select the Manual mode and set the cooking time for 2 minutes on High Pressure. When the timer goes off, do a quick pressure release. Carefully open the lid.

3. Serve hot.

Tomato and Parsley Quinoa Salad

Prep time: 5 minutes | Cook time: 21 minutes | Serves 4

2 tablespoons olive oil

2 cloves garlic, minced

1 cup diced tomatoes

¼ cup chopped fresh Italian flat-leaf parsley

1 tablespoon fresh lemon juice

1 cup quinoa

2 cups water

1 teaspoon salt

1. Press the Sauté button on the Instant Pot and heat the olive oil. Add the garlic and sauté for 30 seconds. Add the tomatoes, parsley and lemon juice. Sauté for an additional minute. Transfer the tomato mixture to a small bowl.

2. Add the quinoa and water to the Instant Pot.

3. Lock the lid. Select the Manual mode and set the cooking time for 20 minutes on High Pressure. Once the timer goes off, perform a natural pressure release for 10 minutes, then release any remaining pressure. Carefully open the lid.

4. Fluff the cooked quinoa with a fork. Stir in the tomato mixture and salt.

5. Serve immediately.

Vanilla Rice Pudding

Prep time: 5 minutes | Cook time: 20 minutes | Serves 4

2 cups whole milk

1¼ cups water

1 teaspoon cinnamon

½ teaspoon grated nutmeg

Pinch of salt

1 cup long-grain rice, rinsed and drained

1 teaspoon vanilla extract

1 can (14-ounce / 397-g) condensed milk

1. Add the whole milk, water, cinnamon, nutmeg and salt into the Instant Pot.

2. Add rice and stir to combine.

3. Lock the lid. Select the Porridge mode and set the cooking time for 20 minutes on High Pressure. Once the timer goes off, perform a natural pressure release for 10 minutes, then release any remaining pressure. Carefully open the lid.

4. Add the vanilla extract and condensed milk. Stir well until creamy and serve.

Vinegary Pearl Onion

Prep time: 5 minutes | Cook time: 5 minutes | Serves 4

1 pound (454 g) pearl onions, peeled

Pinch of salt and black pepper

½ cup water

1 bay leaf

4 tablespoons balsamic vinegar

1 tablespoon coconut flour

1 tablespoon stevia

1. In the pot, mix the pearl onions with salt, pepper, water, and bay leaf.

2. Set the lid in place. Select the Manual mode and set the cooking time for 5 minutes on Low Pressure. When the timer goes off, do a quick pressure release. Carefully open the lid.

3. Meanwhile, in a pan, add the vinegar, stevia, and flour. Mix and bring to a simmer. Remove from the heat. Pour over the pearl onions. Mix and serve.

Watercress Appetizer Salad

Prep time: 12 mins, Cook Time: 2 mins, Servings: 4

- 1 bunch watercress, roughly torn
- ½ cup water
- 1 tbsp. lemon juice
- 1 cubed watermelon
- 1 tbsp. olive oil
- 2 peaches, pitted and sliced

1. In the Instant Pot, mix watercress with water.

2. Lock the lid. Select the Manual mode, then set the timer for 2 minutes at High Pressure.

3. Once the timer goes off, do a quick pressure release. Carefully open the lid.

4. Drain the watercress and transfer to a bowl. Add peaches, watermelon, oil, and lemon juice, and toss well. Divide the salad into salad bowls and serve.

Zucchini Spread

Prep time: 12 mins, Cook Time: 9 mins, Servings: 6

- ½ cup water
- 1 tbsp. olive oil
- 1 bunch basil, chopped
- 1½ lbs. zucchinis, chopped
- 2 garlic cloves, minced

1.   Set the Instant Pot to Sauté and heat the olive oil. Cook the garlic cloves for 3 minutes, stirring occasionally.

2.   Add zucchinis and water, and mix well.

3.   Lock the lid. Select the Manual mode, then set the timer for 3 minutes at High Pressure.

4.   Once the timer goes off, do a quick pressure release. Carefully open the lid.

5.   Add the basil and blend the mixture with an immersion blender until smooth.

6.   Select the Simmer mode and cook for 2 minutes more.

7.   Transfer to a bowl and serve warm.

CHAPTER 13 SIDE DISHES

Sweet-and-Sour Kale and Beets

Prep time: 10 minutes | Cook time: 10 minutes | Serves 6

4 cups quartered beets
3 cups roughly chopped kale
1 cup sliced onion
1½ cups water
¼ cup walnut oil
¼ cup apple cider vinegar
1 tablespoon brown sugar
½ teaspoon salt
1 teaspoon black pepper

1. Combine the beets and the water in the Instant Pot.
2. Set the lid in place. Select the Manual mode and set the cooking time for 5 minutes on High Pressure. When the timer goes off, do a quick pressure release. Carefully open the lid.
3. Add in the kale and the onion.
4. Lock the lid again. Select the Manual mode and set the cooking time for 5 minutes on High Pressure. Once the timer goes off, perform a natural pressure release for 5 minutes, then release any remaining pressure.
5. While the steam is releasing, combine the walnut oil, apple cider vinegar, brown sugar, salt and black pepper. Whisk together until well blended.
6. Carefully open the lid. Remove the vegetables from the pot and thoroughly drain them.
7. Transfer the vegetables to a bowl and add in the dressing. Toss to coat.
8. Serve warm, or cover and refrigerate for several hours for a chilled side dish.

Spaghetti Squash with Olives

Prep time: 15 minutes | Cook time: 10 minutes | Serves 10

1 cup water
1 medium spaghetti squash, halved lengthwise and seeds removed
¼ cup sliced green olives with pimientos
1 can (14-ounce / 397-g) diced tomatoes, drained
1 teaspoon dried oregano
½ teaspoon salt
½ teaspoon pepper
½ cup shredded Cheddar cheese, for serving
¼ cup minced fresh basil, for serving

1. Pour the water into the Instant Pot and insert a trivet. Place the spaghetti squash on top of the trivet.
2. Secure the lid. Select the Manual mode and set the cooking time for 7 minutes at High Pressure.
3. Once cooking is complete, do a quick pressure release. Carefully open the lid.
4. Remove the spaghetti squash and trivet from the Instant Pot. Drain the cooking liquid from the pot.
5. Separate the squash into strands resembling spaghetti with a fork and discard the skin.
6. Return the squash to the Instant Pot. Add the olives, tomatoes, oregano, salt, and pepper and stir to combine.
7. Press the Sauté button on the Instant Pot and cook for about 3 minutes until heated through.
8. Serve topped with the cheese and basil.

Pesto Spaghetti Squash

Prep time: 5 minutes | Cook time: 12 minutes | Serves 6

1½ cups plus 3 tablespoons water, divided
1 (3-pound / 1.4-kg) spaghetti squash, pierced with a knife about 10 times
¼ cup pesto

1. Pour 1½ cups of the water and insert the trivet in the Instant Pot. Put the pan on the trivet. Place the squash on the trivet.
2. Lock the lid. Select the Manual mode and set the cooking time for 12 minutes on High Pressure. Once the timer goes off, perform a natural pressure release for 10 minutes, then release any remaining pressure. Carefully open the lid.
3. Using tongs, carefully transfer the squash to a cutting board to cool for about 10 minutes.
4. Halve the spaghetti squash lengthwise. Using a spoon, scoop out and discard the seeds. Using a fork,

scrape the flesh of the squash and shred into long "noodles". Place the noodles in a medium serving bowl.

5. In a small bowl, mix the pesto with the remaining 3 tablespoons of the water. Drizzle over the squash, toss to combine, and serve warm.

Spiced Orange Carrots

Prep time: 5 minutes | Cook time: 4 to 5 minutes | Serves 6

2 pounds (907 g) medium carrots or baby carrots, cut into ¾-inch pieces

½ cup orange juice

½ cup packed brown sugar

2 tablespoons butter

¾ teaspoon ground cinnamon

¼ teaspoon ground nutmeg

½ teaspoon salt

¼ cup cold water

1 tablespoon cornstarch

1. Mix together all the ingredients except the water and cornstarch in your Instant Pot.

2. Secure the lid. Press the Manual button on your Instant Pot and cook for 3 minutes on Low Pressure.

3. When the timer goes off, use a quick pressure release. Carefully remove the lid.

4. Press the sauté button on your Instant Pot and bring the liquid to a boil. Fold in the water and cornstarch and stir until smooth.

5. Continue to cook for 1 to 2 minutes and stir until the sauce is thickened.

6. Transfer to a serving dish and serve immediately.

Ginger-Garlic Spicy Kale

Prep time: 5 minutes | Cook time: 6 minutes | Serves 4

1 tablespoon olive oil

5 cloves garlic

1 tablespoon fresh grated ginger

1 tablespoon crushed red pepper flakes

8 cups kale, stems removed and chopped

1½ cups vegetable broth

1 tablespoon garlic chili paste

1. Press the Sauté button on the Instant Pot and heat the oil. Add in the garlic, ginger and crushed red pepper flakes. Sauté the mixture for 2 minutes or until highly fragrant.

2. Add in the vegetable broth and garlic chili paste. Whisk until well blended. Add in the kale and stir.

3. Lock the lid. Select the Manual mode and set the cooking time for 4 minutes on High Pressure. Once the timer goes off, perform a natural pressure release for 5 minutes, then release any remaining pressure. Carefully open the lid.

4. Stir before serving.

Spicy Green Beans

Prep time: 5 minutes | Cook time: 3 minutes | Serves 4 to 6

1½ pounds (680 g) green beans, ends trimmed

¼ cup low-sodium soy sauce

¼ cup vegetable or garlic broth

3 cloves garlic, minced

2 tablespoons sriracha

2 tablespoons sesame oil

1 tablespoon paprika

1 tablespoon rice vinegar

2 teaspoons garlic powder

1 teaspoon onion powder

2 tablespoons chopped almonds (optional)

¼ teaspoon crushed red pepper flakes (optional)

¼ teaspoon cayenne pepper (optional)

1. Stir together all the ingredients in the Instant Pot.

2. Lock the lid. Select the Manual mode and set the cooking time for 3 minutes at High Pressure.

3. Once cooking is complete, do a quick pressure release. Carefully open the lid.

4. Serve warm.

Ratatouille

Prep time: 15 minutes | Cook time: 8 minutes | Serves 6

1 (1-pound / 454-g) globe eggplant, cut into 1-inch pieces

3 zucchinis, cut into 1-inch pieces

1 teaspoon fine sea salt

2 tablespoons extra-virgin olive oil, plus more for serving

1 large yellow onion, cut into 1-inch pieces

2 cloves garlic, minced

1 teaspoon dried basil

½ teaspoon freshly ground black pepper

½ teaspoon dried thyme

½ teaspoon red pepper flakes

1 bay leaf

3 red bell peppers, stemmed, deseeded and cut into 1-inch pieces

1 (14½-ounce / 411-g) can diced tomatoes

¼ cup dry white wine

Fresh basil leaves, for serving

Crusty bread, for serving

1. In a large bowl, toss together the eggplant and zucchini with the salt. Let stand for 15 minutes.
2. Select the Sauté setting on the Instant Pot, add the oil, and heat for 1 minute. Add the onion and garlic and sauté for about 4 minutes, or until the onion softens. Add the basil, black pepper, thyme, red pepper flakes, and bay leaf and sauté for about 1 minute. Add the eggplant-zucchini mixture and any liquid that has pooled in the bottom of the bowl, along with the bell peppers, tomatoes and their liquid, and wine. Stir to combine.
3. Set the lid in place. Select the Manual mode and set the cooking time for 2 minutes on Low Pressure. When the timer goes off, do a quick pressure release. Carefully open the lid.
4. Discard the bay leaf. Spoon the ratatouille into a serving bowl.
5. Drizzle the ratatouille with oil and sprinkle with fresh basil. Serve warm, with crusty bread.

Sriracha Collard Greens

Prep time: 10 minutes | Cook time: 10 minutes | Serves 6

2 pounds (907 g) collard greens, washed, spines removed, and chopped

1 cup chicken broth

1 small onion, peeled and diced

¼ cup apple cider vinegar

1 slice bacon

1 teaspoon sriracha

½ teaspoon sea salt

¼ teaspoon ground black pepper

1. Combine all the ingredients in Instant Pot.
2. Secure the lid. Select the Manual mode and set the cooking time for 10 minutes at High Pressure.
3. Once cooking is complete, do a natural pressure release for 10 minutes, then release any remaining pressure. Carefully open the lid.
4. Discard the bacon and transfer the collard greens to a bowl. Serve immediately.

Steamed Artichoke with Aioli Sauce

Prep time: 10 minutes | Cook time: 15 minutes | Serves 2

1 large artichoke

1 cup water

Juice of ½ lemon

The Aioli Dipping Sauce:

½ cup raw cashews, soaked overnight or 2 hours in hot water

1½ tablespoons Dijon mustard

1 tablespoon apple cider vinegar

Juice of ½ lemon

2 cloves garlic

Pinch of ground turmeric

½ teaspoon sea salt

⅓ cup water

1. Fit the inner pot with the trivet and add 1 cup water. Trim the artichoke stem so that it is 1 to 2 inches long, and trim about 1 inch off the top. Squeeze the lemon juice over the top of the artichoke and add the lemon rind to the water. Place the artichoke, top-side down, on the trivet.
2. Set the lid in place. Select the Steam mode and set the cooking time for 15 minutes on High Pressure. When the timer goes off, do a quick pressure release. Carefully open the lid.
3. Check for doneness. Leaves should be easy to remove and the "meat" at the base of each leaf should be tender.
4. Meanwhile, make the aioli dipping sauce. Drain the cashews and place them in a blender. Add the Dijon, vinegar, lemon juice, garlic, turmeric, and sea salt. Add

half the water and blend. Continue adding water as you blend until the sauce is smooth and creamy. Transfer the sauce to a small bowl or jar. Refrigerate until ready to use.

5. Use tongs to remove the hot artichoke and place on a serving dish. Serve the artichoke warm with the aioli.

Zucchini and Chickpea Tagine

Prep time: 30 minutes | Cook time: 5 minutes | Serves 12

2 tablespoons olive oil

2 garlic cloves, minced

2 teaspoons paprika

1 teaspoon ground cumin

1 teaspoon ground ginger

½ teaspoon salt

¼ teaspoon ground cinnamon

¼ teaspoon pepper

2 medium zucchini, cut into ½-inch pieces

1 small butternut squash, peeled and cut into ½-inch cubes

1 can (15-ounce / 425-g) chickpeas or garbanzo beans, rinsed and drained

12 dried apricots, halved

½ cup water

1 medium sweet red pepper, coarsely chopped

1 medium onion, coarsely chopped

2 teaspoon honey

2 to 3 teaspoon harissa chili paste

1 can (14.5-ounce / 411-g) crushed tomatoes, undrained

¼ cup chopped fresh mint leaves

1. Press the Sauté button on the Instant Pot and heat the olive oil until it shimmers.

2. Add the garlic, paprika, cumin, ginger, salt, cinnamon, and pepper and cook for about 1 minute until fragrant. Add the remaining ingredients except the tomatoes and mint to the Instant Pot and stir to combine.

3. Secure the lid. Select the Manual mode and set the cooking time for 3 minutes at High Pressure.

4. Once cooking is complete, do a quick pressure release. Carefully open the lid.

5. Stir in the tomatoes and mint until heated though. Serve warm.

Zucchini-Parmesan Cheese Fritters

Prep time: 15 minutes | Cook time: 24 minutes | Serves 4

4 cups shredded zucchini

1 teaspoon salt

⅓ cup shredded Parmesan cheese

⅓ cup all-purpose flour

1 large egg, beaten

2 cloves garlic, minced

½ teaspoon black pepper

6 tablespoons olive oil, plus more as needed

1. In a colander, add the zucchini and lightly sprinkle with the salt. Let stand for 10 minutes.

2. Remove from the colander and pat the zucchini dry using a paper towel to gently press as much moisture out as you can.

3. In a large bowl, mix together the zucchini, Parmesan, flour, egg, garlic, and pepper and stir well.

4. Press the Sauté button on the Instant Pot. Add 2 tablespoons of the oil into the pot.

5. Working in batches, scoop out tablespoonfuls of the zucchini mixture and add to the Instant Pot, pressing down gently with the back of a spoon to create 2½ rounds.

6. Cook for 4 minutes per side until lightly browned on both sides.

7. Remove the zucchini fitters with a slotted spatula. Repeat with the remaining zucchini mixture, adding more oil, if needed, with each batch.

8. Allow to cool for 5 minutes before serving.

CHAPTER 14 SAUCE AND BROTH

Marinara Sauce

Prep time: 5 minutes | Cook time: 13 minutes | Makes 4 cups

2 tablespoons oil
1 medium onion, grated
3 garlic cloves, roughly chopped
1 (28-ounce / 794-g) can or carton whole or crushed tomatoes
1 teaspoon kosher salt, plus more as needed
Freshly ground black pepper, to taste
½ teaspoon dried oregano or 2 oregano sprigs
Pinch granulated or raw sugar (optional)

1. Press the Sauté button on the Instant Pot and heat the oil until it shimmers.
2. Add the grated onion and sauté for 2 minutes until tender. Add the garlic and sauté for 1 minute.
3. Fold in the tomatoes, salt, oregano, and pepper and stir well.
4. Secure the lid. Select the Manual mode and set the cooking time for 10 minutes at High Pressure.
5. Once cooking is complete, do a quick pressure release. Carefully open the lid.
6. Taste and adjust the seasoning, if needed. Add the sugar to balance the acidity of the tomatoes, if desired.
7. Store in an airtight container in the refrigerator for up to 4 days or freeze for up to 6 months.

Carrot and Mushroom Broth

Prep time: 10 minutes | Cook time: 20 minutes | Makes 8 cups

4 medium carrots, peeled and cut into large pieces
2 large leeks, trimmed and cut into large pieces
2 large yellow onions, peeled and quartered
1 large stalk celery, chopped
2 cups sliced button mushrooms
5 whole cloves garlic
Pinch of dried red pepper flakes
8½ cups water

1. Add all the ingredients to the Instant Pot and stir to combine.

2. Lock the lid. Select the Manual mode and set the cooking time for 20 minutes on High Pressure. Once the timer goes off, perform a natural pressure release for 15 minutes, then release any remaining pressure. Carefully open the lid.
3. Strain the broth through a fine-mesh strainer or through cheesecloth placed in a colander.
4. Store in a covered container in the refrigerator or freezer.

Corn and Mushroom Stock

Prep time: 10 minutes | Cook time: 15 minutes | Serves 8

4 large mushrooms, diced
2 cobs of corns
1 small onion, unpeeled and halved
1 celery stalk, chopped into thirds
1 teaspoon dried bay leaf
1 teaspoon grated ginger
1 sprig fresh parsley
1 teaspoon kosher salt
½ teaspoon ground turmeric
½ teaspoon whole black peppercorns
8 cups water

1. Place all the ingredients into the Instant Pot and stir well.
2. Lock the lid. Press the Manual button on the Instant Pot and set the cooking time for 15 minutes at High Pressure.
3. Once cooking is complete, do a natural pressure release for 10 minutes, then release any remaining pressure. Carefully open the lid.
4. Strain the stock through a fine-mesh strainer and discard all the solids.
5. Serve immediately or refrigerate in an airtight container for 3 to 4 days.

Mushroom Broth

Prep time: 5 minutes | Cook time: 15 minutes | Serves 8

4 ounces (113 g) dried mushrooms, soaked and rinsed

½ cup celery, chopped

½ cup carrots, chopped

4 cloves garlic, crushed

4 bay leaves

1 onion, quartered

8 cups water

Salt and ground black pepper, to taste.

1. Add all the ingredients except the salt and pepper to the Instant Pot and stir well.
2. Lock the lid. Press the Manual button on the Instant Pot and set the cooking time for 15 minutes at High Pressure.
3. Once cooking is complete, do a quick pressure release. Open the lid.
4. Add the salt and pepper to taste.
5. Over a large bowl, carefully strain the stock through a fine-mesh strainer. Discard all the solids.
6. Serve immediately or store in a sealed container in the refrigerator for 4 to 5 days or in the freezer for up to 6 months.

Pork and Carrot Broth

Prep time: 5 minutes | Cook time: 1 hour | Serves 8

3 pounds (1.4 kg) pork bones

3 large carrots, cut into large chunks

3 large stalks celery, cut into large chunks

2 cloves garlic, sliced

1 bay leaf

1 tablespoon apple cider vinegar

8 cups water

1 teaspoon whole peppercorns

Salt, to taste

1. Place all the ingredients into the Instant Pot and stir to incorporate.
2. Secure the lid. Select the Manual mode and set the cooking time for 1 hour at High Pressure.
3. When the timer beeps, perform a natural pressure release for 10 minutes, then release any remaining pressure. Carefully remove the lid.
4. Allow the broth to cool for 10 to 15 minutes. Strain the broth through a fine-mesh strainer and discard all the solids.
5. Serve immediately or store in a sealed container in the refrigerator for 4 to 5 days or in the freezer for up to 6 months.

Ranch Dip

Prep time: 6 mins, Cook Time: 2 mins, Servings: 8

- 1 cup olive oil
- Salt and pepper, to taste
- 1 cup beaten egg whites
- 1 tsp. mustard paste
- Juice of 1 lemon

1. In the Instant Pot, add all the ingredients and mix well.
2. Press the Sauté button and heat for 2 minutes while stirring. Do not bring to a simmer.
3. You can serve the ranch dip with chicken nuggets, French fries, or green salad.

Satay Sauce

Prep time: 6 mins, Cook Time: 3 hours, Servings: 6

- ⅓ cup peanut butter
- 1 red chili pepper, finely chopped
- 4 tbsps. soy sauce
- 1 cup coconut milk
- 1 garlic clove, minced

1. Place all ingredients in the Instant Pot and stir until everything is well combined.
2. Lock the lid. Select the Slow Cook mode, then set the timer for 3 hours at High Pressure.
3. Once the timer goes off, do a quick pressure release. Carefully open the lid.
4. Serve the satay sauce with beef kebabs or chicken skewers, or you can serve it as dipping sauce.

Seafood Stock

Prep time: 5 minutes | Cook time: 30 minutes | Serves 8

8 cups water

Shells and heads from ½ pound (227 g) prawns

3 cloves garlic, sliced

4 carrots, cut into chunks

4 onions, quartered

2 bay leaves

1 teaspoon whole black peppercorns

1. Place all the ingredients into the Instant Pot.
2. Secure the lid. Select the Manual mode and set the cooking time for 30 minutes at High Pressure.
3. Once cooking is complete, do a natural pressure release for 15 minutes, then release any remaining pressure. Remove the lid.
4. Over a large bowl, carefully strain the stock through a fine-mesh strainer.
5. Serve immediately or store in an airtight container in the refrigerator for 3 days or in the freezer for up to 3 months.

Almond Milk

Prep time: 5 minutes | Cook time: 10 minutes | Makes 4 cups

1 cup almonds

6 cups water, divided

1. Add the almonds and 2 cups of the water to the Instant Pot.
2. Lock the lid. Select the Manual mode and set the cooking time for 10 minutes on High Pressure.
3. Once the timer goes off, perform a natural pressure release for 10 minutes, then release any remaining pressure. Carefully open the lid. Drain the almonds.
4. In a blender, combine the almonds and 4 cups of the water and blend well. Strain through a nut milk bag and store in the refrigerator.

Thousand Island Dressing

Prep time: 10 mins, Cook Time: 2 hours, Servings: 4

- 1 tsp. tabasco
- 1 shallot, finely chopped
- 1 cup mayonnaise
- 4 tbsps. chopped dill pickles
- 1 tbsp. freshly squeezed lemon juice
- ¼ cup water
- Salt and pepper, to taste

1. Place all the ingredients in the Instant Pot and whisk to combine.
2. Lock the lid. Select the Slow Cook mode, then set the timer for 2 hours at High Pressure.
3. Once the timer goes off, do a quick pressure release. Carefully open the lid.
4. You can use this dressing to serve the burgers, sandwiches, or salads.

Caramel Sauce

Prep time: 5 minutes | Cook time: 45 minutes | Serves 4 to 6

1 (11-ounce / 312-g) can sweetened condensed coconut milk

1 cup water

1 teaspoon coarse sea salt (optional)

1. Peel the label off the can and place the can on a trivet and into your Instant Pot. Pour in the water.
2. Lock the lid. Select the Manual mode and set the cooking time for 45 minutes on High Pressure. Once the timer goes off, perform a natural pressure release for 20 minutes, then release any remaining pressure. Carefully open the lid.
3. Remove the can and trivet. Set aside until cool enough to handle.
4. Once cooled, open the can and pour the caramel sauce into a glass jar for storage. For a salted caramel, stir in the sea salt.

Tabasco Sauce

Prep time: 5 minutes | Cook time: 1 hour | Makes 2 cups

18 ounces (510 g) fresh hot peppers or any kind, stems removed and chopped

1¾ cups apple cider

3 teaspoons smoked or plain salt

1. Combine all the ingredients in the Instant Pot.

2. Lock the lid. Press the Manual button on the Instant Pot and set the cooking time for 1 hour at High Pressure.

3. Once cooking is complete, do a natural pressure release for 15 minutes, then release any remaining pressure. Carefully open the lid.

4. Purée the mixture with an immersion blender until smooth.

5. Serve immediately or refrigerate until ready to use.

Basil Tomato Sauce

Prep time: 5 minutes | Cook time: 16 minutes | Serves 4

1 tablespoon olive oil

3 cloves garlic, minced

2½ pounds (1.1 kg) Roma tomatoes, diced

½ cup chopped basil

¼ cup vegetable broth

Salt, to taste

1. Set your Instant Pot to Sauté and heat the olive oil.

2. Add the minced garlic and sauté for 1 minute until fragrant. Stir in the tomatoes, basil, and vegetable broth.

3. Lock the lid. Press the Manual button on the Instant Pot and cook for 10 minutes at High Pressure.

4. Once cooking is complete, do a quick pressure release. Carefully open the lid.

5. Set your Instant Pot to Sauté again and cook for another 5 minutes.

6. Blend the mixture with an immersion blender until smooth.

7. Season with salt to taste. Serve chilled or at room temperature.

Tomato Salsa

Prep time: 10 minutes | Cook time: 30 minutes | Serves 6

6 cups fresh tomatoes, diced, peeled, and deseeded

1½ (6-ounce / 170-g) cans tomato paste

1½ green bell peppers, diced

1 cup jalapeño peppers, deseeded and chopped

¼ cup vinegar

2 yellow onions, diced

½ tablespoon kosher salt

1½ tablespoons sugar

1 tablespoon cayenne pepper

1 tablespoon garlic powder

1. Place all the ingredients into the Instant Pot and stir to incorporate.

2. Secure the lid. Select the Manual mode and set the cooking time for 30 minutes at High Pressure.

3. Once cooking is complete, do a natural pressure release for 10 minutes, then release any remaining pressure. Carefully open the lid.

4. Serve immediately or refrigerate in an airtight container for up to 5 days.

Cinnamon-Vanilla Applesauce

Prep time: 10 minutes | Cook time: 5 minutes | Serves 6 to 8

3 pounds (1.4 kg) apples, cored and quartered

⅓ cup water

1 teaspoon ground cinnamon

1 teaspoon freshly squeezed lemon juice

1 teaspoon vanilla extract

½ teaspoon salt

1. Add all the ingredients to the Instant Pot and stir to combine.

2. Lock the lid. Select the Manual mode and set the cooking time for 5 minutes on High Pressure. Once the timer goes off, perform a natural pressure release for 10 minutes, then release any remaining pressure. Carefully open the lid.

3. Using an immersion blender, blend the applesauce until smooth.

4. Serve immediately or refrigerate until ready to use.

Vegetable Stock

Prep time: 5 minutes | Cook time: 30 minutes | Serves 8

8 cups water

4 celery stalks, cut into chunks

4 carrots, cut into chunks

4 thyme sprigs

6 parsley sprigs

2 teaspoons chopped garlic

2 bay leaves

2 green onions, sliced

10 whole black peppercorns

1½ teaspoons salt

1.   Except for the salt, add all the ingredients to the Instant Pot.

2.   Secure the lid. Select the Soup mode and set the cooking time for 30 minutes at High Pressure.

3.   Once cooking is complete, do a natural pressure release for 15 minutes, then release any remaining pressure. Remove the lid.

4.   Sprinkle with the salt and whisk well.

5.   Over a large bowl, carefully strain the stock through a fine-mesh strainer.

6.   Serve immediately or store in an airtight container in the refrigerator for 4 to 5 days or in the freezer for up to 3 months.

CHAPTER 15 DESSERTS

Chocolate Almond Fudge

Prep time: 5 minutes | Cook time: 5 minutes | Serves 30

2½ cups Swerve

1¾ cups unsweetened almond milk

1½ cups almond butter

8 ounces (227 g) unsweetened baking chocolate, finely chopped

1 teaspoon almond or vanilla extract

¼ teaspoon fine sea salt

1. Line a baking dish with greased parchment paper.

2. Place the sweetener, almond milk, almond butter, and chocolate in the Instant Pot. Stir well. Select the Sauté mode and cook for 2 minutes.

3. Set the Instant Pot to Keep Warm for 3 minutes, or until the fudge mixture is completely melted and well mixed. Fold in the extract and salt and stir well.

4. Pour the fudge mixture into the prepared baking dish, cover, and refrigerate until firm, about 4 hours.

5. Cut the fudge into 30 equal-sized pieces and serve.

Apple and Oatmeal Crisps

Prep time: 15 minutes | Cook time: 5 minutes | Serves 4

5 apples, cored and chopped

1 tablespoon honey

2 teaspoons cinnamon powder

½ teaspoon nutmeg powder

1 cup water

¾ cup old fashioned rolled oats

¼ cup all-purpose flour

4 tablespoons unsalted butter, melted

½ teaspoon salt

¼ cup brown sugar

1 cup vanilla ice cream, for topping

1. In the Instant Pot, mix the apples, honey, cinnamon, nutmeg, and water.

2. In a medium bowl, combine the rolled oats, flour, butter, salt, and brown sugar. Drizzle the mixture over the apples.

3. Seal the lid, set to the Manual mode and set the cooking time for 5 minutes on High Pressure.

4. When cooking is complete, allow a natural pressure release for 10 minutes, then release any remaining pressure. Carefully open the lid.

5. Spoon the apple into serving bowls, top with vanilla ice cream and serve immediately.

Apple Bread

Prep time: 12 mins, Cook Time: 1 hour, Servings: 4

- 1 tbsp. baking powder
- 3 eggs
- 1½ cups sweetened condensed milk
- 2½ cups white flour
- 3 apples, peeled, cored and chopped
- 1 tbsp. melted coconut oil
- 1 cup water

1. In a bowl, mix the baking powder with eggs and whisk well.

2. Add the milk, flour and apple pieces, whisk well and pour into a loaf pan greased with coconut oil.

3. In the Instant Pot, add the water. Arrange a trivet in the pot, then place the loaf pan on the trivet.

4. Lock the lid. Set the Instant Pot to Slow Cook mode, then set the timer for 1 hour at High Pressure.

5. When the timer goes off, perform a natural release for 10 minutes, then release any remaining pressure. Carefully open the lid.

6. Leave apple bread to cool down, slice and serve.

Apple Wontons

Prep time: 10 minutes | Cook time: 12 minutes | Serves 8

1 (8-ounce / 227-g) can refrigerated crescent rolls

1 large apple, peeled, cored, and cut into 8 wedges

4 tablespoons unsalted butter

2 teaspoons ground cinnamon

¼ teaspoon ground nutmeg

½ cup brown sugar

1 teaspoon vanilla extract

¾ cup orange juice

1. Make the dumplings: Unfold the crescent rolls on a clean work surface, then separate into the 8 triangles.

Place 1 apple wedge on each crescent roll triangle and fold the dough around the apple to enclose it. Set aside.

2. Select the Sauté mode of the Instant Pot. Add the butter and heat for 2 minutes until melted.

3. Add the cinnamon, nutmeg, sugar, and vanilla, heating and stirring until melted.

4. Place the dumplings in the Instant Pot and mix in the orange juice.

5. Lock the lid. Select the Manual mode. Set the time for 10 minutes at High Pressure.

6. When cooking is complete, let the pressure release naturally for 5 minutes, then release any remaining pressure. Unlock the lid.

7. Serve immediately.

Apricots Dulce de Leche

Prep time: 15 minutes | Cook time: 25 minutes | Serves 6

5 cups water
2 cups sweetened condensed milk
4 apricots, halved, cored, and sliced

1. Pour the water in the Instant Pot and fit in a trivet. Divide condensed milk into 6 medium jars and close with lids. Place jars on trivet.

2. Seal the lid, set to the Manual mode and set the timer for 25 minutes at High Pressure.

3. When cooking is complete, use a natural pressure release for 10 minutes, then release any remaining pressure. Unlock the lid.

4. Use a fork to whisk until creamy. Serve with sliced apricots.

Beer Poached Pears

Prep time: 5 minutes | Cook time: 10 minutes | Serves 2
3 peeled (stem on) firm pears
1½ cups (1 bottle) stout beer
½ cup packed brown sugar
1 vanilla bean, split lengthwise and seeds scraped

1. Slice a thin layer from the bottom of each pear so they can stand upright. Use a melon baller to scoop out the seeds and core from the bottom.

2. Stir together the beer, brown sugar, and vanilla bean and seeds in the Instant Pot until combined. Place the pears upright in the pot.

3. Lock the lid. Select the Manual mode and set the cooking time for 9 minutes at High Pressure.

4. When the timer beeps, perform a quick pressure release. Carefully remove the lid.

5. Using tongs, carefully remove the pears by their stems and transfer to a plate and set aside.

6. Set the Instant Pot to Sauté and simmer until the liquid in the Instant Pot is reduced by half.

7. Strain the liquid into a bowl through a fine-mesh sieve, then pour over the pears.

8. Serve at room temperature or chilled.

Oat and Black Bean Brownies

Prep time: 5 minutes | Cook time: 25 minutes | Serves 4
1½ cups canned black beans, drained
½ cup steel-cut oats
½ teaspoon salt
3 tablespoons unsweetened cocoa powder
½ cup maple syrup
¼ cup coconut oil
¾ teaspoon baking powder
½ cup chocolate chips
Cooking spray
1½ cups water

1. Pulse the black beans, oats, salt, cocoa powder, maple syrup, coconut oil, and baking powder in a food processor until very smooth.

2. Pour the batter into a medium bowl and fold in the chocolate chips.

3. Spray a 7-inch springform pan with cooking spray and pour in the batter. Cover the pan with aluminum foil.

4. Pour the water into the Instant Pot and insert a trivet. Place the pan on the trivet.

5. Lock the lid. Select the Manual mode and set the cooking time for 25 minutes at High Pressure.

6. When the timer beeps, perform a natural pressure release for 10 minutes, then release any remaining pressure. Carefully remove the lid.

7. Let cool for 5 minutes, then transfer to the fridge to chill for 1 to 2 hours.

8. Cut the brownies into squares and serve.

Bourbon and Date Pudding Cake

Prep time: 15 minutes | Cook time: 25 minutes | Serves 4

¾ cup all-purpose flour

¼ teaspoon allspice

½ teaspoon baking soda

¼ teaspoon cloves powder

½ teaspoon cinnamon powder

¼ teaspoon salt

1 teaspoon baking powder

2 tablespoons bourbon

3 tablespoons unsalted butter, melted

6 tablespoons hot water

2 tablespoons whole milk

1 egg, beaten

½ cup chopped dates

1 cup water

½ cup caramel sauce

1. In a bowl, combine the flour, allspice, baking soda, cloves, cinnamon, salt, and baking powder.

2. In another bowl, mix the bourbon, butter, hot water, and milk. Pour the bourbon mixture into the flour mixture and mix until well mixed. Whisk in egg and fold in dates.

3. Spritz 4 medium ramekins with cooking spray. Divide the mixture among them, and cover with foil.

4. Pour the water in the Instant Pot, then fit in a trivet and place ramekins on top.

5. Seal the lid, select the Manual mode and set the cooking time for 25 minutes at High Pressure.

6. When cooking is complete, perform a natural pressure release for 10 minutes, then release any remaining pressure.

7. Unlock the lid and carefully remove ramekins, invert onto plates, and drizzle caramel sauce on top. Serve warm.

Coconut Brown Rice Pudding

Prep time: 15 minutes | Cook time: 22 minutes | Serves 6

1 cup long-grain brown rice, rinsed

2 cups water

1 (15-ounce / 425-g) can full-fat coconut milk

½ teaspoon pure vanilla extract

½ teaspoon ground cinnamon

⅓ cup maple syrup

Pinch fine sea salt

1. Combine the rice and water in the Instant Pot and secure the lid. Select the Manual mode and set the cooking time for 22 minutes on Low Pressure.

2. When timer beeps, allow the pressure to naturally release for 10 minutes, then release any remaining pressure. Carefully open the lid.

3. Add the coconut milk, vanilla, cinnamon, maple syrup, and salt. Stir well to combine.

4. Use an immersion blender to pulse the pudding until creamy. Serve warm or you can refrigerate the pudding for an hour before serving.

Bulletproof Hot Choco

Prep time: 6 mins, Cook Time: 5 mins, Servings: 1

- 2 tbsps. coconut oil, divided
- ½ cup coconut milk
- ½ cup water
- 2 tbsps. unsweetened cocoa powder
- Dash of cinnamon
- 1 tsp. erythritol

1. Place 1 tablespoon of coconut oil and milk in the Instant Pot and pour in the water.

2. Lock the lid. Set the Instant Pot to Manual mode, then set the timer for 5 minutes at High Pressure.

3. When the timer goes off, perform a quick release.

4. Open the lid and press the Sauté button.

5. Add 1 tablespoon of coconut oil, cocoa powder, cinnamon and erythritol. Stir to combine well and the mixture has a thick consistency.

6. Transfer the mixture on a baking sheet, then put the sheet in the refrigerator for several hours. Serve chilled.

Caramel Apple Cobbler

Prep time: 30 minutes | Cook time: 2 minutes | Serves 4

5 apples, cored, peeled, and cut into 1-inch cubes, at room temperature
2 tablespoons caramel syrup
½ teaspoon ground nutmeg
2 teaspoons ground cinnamon
2 tablespoons maple syrup
½ cup water
¾ cup old-fashioned oats
¼ cup all-purpose flour
⅓ cup brown sugar
4 tablespoons salted butter, softened
½ teaspoon sea salt
Vanilla ice cream, for serving

1. Place the apples in the Instant Pot and top with the caramel syrup, nutmeg, cinnamon, maple syrup, and water. Stir to coat well.
2. Combine the oats, flour, brown sugar, butter and salt in a large bowl. Mix well and pour over the apple mixture in the pot.
3. Secure the lid, then select the Manual mode and set the cooking time for 2 minutes on High Pressure.
4. When cooking is complete, perform a natural pressure release for 20minutes, then release any remaining pressure. Carefully open the lid.
5. Transfer the cobbler to a plate, then topped with vanilla ice cream and serve.

Caramel Popcorns

Prep time: 5 minutes | Cook time: 7 minutes | Serves 4

4 tablespoons butter
1 cup sweet corn kernels
3 tablespoons brown sugar
¼ cup whole milk

1. Set the Instant Pot to Sauté mode, melt butter and mix in the corn kernels, heat for 1 minute or until the corn is popping.
2. Cover the lid, and keep cooking for 3 more minutes or until the corn stops popping. Open the lid and transfer the popcorns to a bowl.

3. Combine brown sugar and milk in the pot and cook for 3 minutes or until sugar dissolves. Stir constantly.
4. Drizzle caramel sauce over corns and toss to coat thoroughly. Serve warm.

Cardamom and Pistachio Rice Pudding

Prep time: 15 minutes | Cook time: 10 minutes | Makes 4 cups

½ cup long-grain basmati rice
1½ cups water
1 (13.5-ounce / 383-g) can coconut milk
1 small (5¼-ounce / 149-g) can coconut cream
½ cup brown rice syrup or agave nectar
½ teaspoon ground cardamom
¼ teaspoon fine sea salt
¼ cup currants
¼ cup chopped pistachios

1. Combine the rice and water in the Instant Pot. Secure the lid. Select Manual mode and set the cooking time for 5 minutes at High Pressure.
2. Meanwhile, in a blender, combine the coconut milk, coconut cream, brown rice syrup, cardamom, and salt. Blend at medium speed for about 30 seconds, until smooth. Set aside.
3. When timer beeps, let the pressure release naturally for 10 minutes, then release any remaining pressure. Open the pot and use a whisk to break up the cooked rice. Whisking constantly, pour the coconut milk mixture in a thin stream into the rice.
4. Select the Sauté setting. Cook the pudding for about 5 minutes, whisking constantly, until it is thickened and bubbling.
5. Sit the pudding until set. Remove the pudding from the pot. Stir in the currants.
6. Pour the pudding into a glass or ceramic dish or into individual serving bowls. Cover and refrigerate the pudding for at least 4 hours.
7. Sprinkle the pudding with chopped pistachios. Serve chilled.

Cardamom Yogurt Pudding

Prep time: 20 minutes | Cook time: 15 minutes | Serves 4

1½ cups Greek yogurt

1 teaspoon cocoa powder

2 cups sweetened condensed milk

1 teaspoon cardamom powder

1 cup water

¼ cup mixed nuts, chopped

1. Spritz 4 medium ramekins with cooking spray. Set aside.
2. In a bowl, combine the Greek yogurt, cocoa powder, condensed milk, and cardamom powder. Pour mixture into ramekins and cover with foil.
3. Pour the water into the Instant Pot, then fit in a trivet, and place ramekins on top.
4. Seal the lid, select the Manual mode and set the cooking time for 15 minutes at High Pressure.
5. When cooking is complete, perform a natural pressure release for 15 minutes, then release any remaining pressure. Unlock the lid.
6. Remove the ramekins from the pot, then take off the foil. Top with mixed nuts and serve immediately.

Carrot Raisin Halwa

Prep time: 10 minutes | Cook time: 14 minutes | Serves 6

2 tablespoons coconut oil

2 tablespoons raw cashews

2 tablespoons raisins

2 cups shredded carrots

1 cup almond milk

¼ cup sugar

2 tablespoons ground cashews

¼ teaspoon ground cardamom

Chopped pistachios, for garnish

1. Set the Instant Pot to Sauté and melt the coconut oil until it shimmers.
2. Add the cashews and raisins and cook them until the cashews are golden brown, about 4 minutes.
3. Add the carrots, milk, sugar, and ground cashews, and stir to incorporate.
4. Lock the lid. Select the Manual mode and set the cooking time for 10 minutes at High Pressure.
5. When the timer beeps, perform a natural pressure release for 10 minutes, then release any remaining pressure. Carefully remove the lid.
6. Stir well, mashing the carrots together a bit. Set the Instant Pot to Sauté again and cook, stirring, for about 2 to 3 minutes, until thickened.
7. Turn off the Instant Pot. Stir in the cardamom and let the mixture sit for 10 minutes to thicken up.
8. Garnish with the pistachios and serve.

Simple Chocolate Cake

Prep time: 12 mins, Cook Time: 6 mins, Servings: 3

- 4 tbsps. self-raising flour
- 1 egg
- 4 tbsps. sugar
- 4 tbsps. milk
- 1 tbsp. cocoa powder
- 1 tbsp. melted coconut oil
- 1 cup water

1. In a bowl, combine the flour, egg, sugar, milk and cocoa powder, stir well and set the mixture to a cake pan greased with coconut oil.
2. Add the water to the Instant Pot, add steamer basket, add cake inside.
3. Lock the lid. Set the Instant Pot to Manual mode, then set the timer for 6 minutes at High Pressure.
4. When the timer goes off, perform a natural release for 5 minutes, then release any remaining pressure. Carefully open the lid.
5. Serve the cake warm.

Super Chocolate Cookies

Prep time: 5 minutes | Cook time: 6 minutes | Serves 8

2 cups blanched almond flour

3 tablespoons arrowroot starch

1 teaspoon baking soda

¼ teaspoon sea salt

4 tablespoons melted coconut oil

2 tablespoons pure maple syrup

1 teaspoon pure vanilla extract

⅓ cup chopped dairy-free dark chocolate

1 cup water

1. In a medium bowl, whisk together the almond flour, arrowroot, baking soda, and salt.

2. Make a well in the middle of the dry ingredients. Pour the coconut oil, maple syrup, and vanilla into the well, and whisk to combine.

3. Stir in the dark chocolate. The mixture may be a little crumbly but should hold together when pressed.

4. Cut out a piece of parchment paper to fit the bottom of a springform pan. Press the dough firmly on top of the parchment. Cover the pan with foil.

5. Fit the Instant Pot with a trivet and add the water. Place the foil-covered springform pan onto the trivet.

6. Lock the lid. Select Manual mode and set the cook time for 6 minutes on High Pressure.

7. Once the cook time is complete, allow the pressure to release naturally for 6 minutes, then quick release any remaining pressure.

8. Preheat the oven broiler.

9. Carefully remove the lid and take the pan out of the Instant Pot. Remove the sides of the springform pan.

10. Transfer the cookie under the broiler for 1 minute, or just until golden on top. Let the cookie cool for 10 minutes, then cut into 8 wedges and serve.

Almond Bread

Prep time: 12 mins, Cook Time: 5 hours, Servings: 10

- 1½ tsps. baking powder
- 1½ cups erythritol
- 3 eggs, beaten
- 2½ cups all-purpose flour
- ¼ cup olive oil
- Salt, to taste

1. Mix all ingredients in a mixing bowl.

2. Once properly mixed, pour the batter in the greased Instant Pot.

3. Lock the lid. Set the Instant Pot to Slow Cook mode, then set the timer for 5 hours at High Pressure.

4. When the timer goes off, perform a natural release for 10 minutes, then release any remaining pressure. Carefully open the lid.

5. Serve immediately.

Keto Brownies

Prep time: 12 mins, Cook Time: 5 hours, Servings: 9

- 2 tsps. erythritol
- ¼ cup all-purpose flour
- ½ cup coconut oil
- ⅓ cup dark chocolate chips
- 5 beaten eggs
- Salt, to taste
- 2 tbsps. olive oil

1. Place all the ingredients in a mixing bowl, except for the olive oil.

2. Make sure they are well combined.

3. Grese the Instant Pot with olive oil. Pour the mixture into the greased Instant Pot.

4. Lock the lid. Set the Instant Pot to Slow Cook mode, then set the timer for 5 hours at High Pressure.

5. When the timer goes off, perform a natural release for 10 minutes, then release any remaining pressure. Carefully open the lid.

6. Transfer the brownies on a platter and slice to serve.

Maple Syrup Lemon Pudding

Prep time: 12 mins, Cook Time: 5 mins, Servings: 7

- ½ cup maple syrup
- 3 cups milk
- Lemon zest from 2 grated lemons
- 2 tbsps. gelatin
- Juice of 2 lemons
- 1 cup water

1. In the blender, mix milk with lemon juice, lemon zest, maple syrup and gelatin, pulse really well and divide into ramekins.

2. In the Instant Pot, set in the water, add steamer basket, add ramekins inside.

3. Lock the lid. Set the Instant Pot to Manual mode, then set the timer for 5 minutes on High Pressure.

4. When the timer goes off, perform a natural release. Carefully open the lid.

5. Refrigerate and serve the puddings chilled.

Lemon and Ricotta Torte

Prep time: 15 minutes | Cook time: 35 minutes | Serves 12

Cooking spray

Torte:

1⅓ cups Swerve

½ cup (1 stick) unsalted butter, softened

2 teaspoons lemon or vanilla extract

5 large eggs, separated

2½ cups blanched almond flour

1¼ (10-ounce / 284-g) cups whole-milk ricotta cheese

¼ cup lemon juice

1 cup cold water

Lemon Glaze:

½ cup (1 stick) unsalted butter

¼ cup Swerve

2 tablespoons lemon juice

2 ounces (57 g) cream cheese (¼ cup)

Grated lemon zest and lemon slices, for garnish

1. Line a baking pan with parchment paper and spray with cooking spray. Set aside.
2. Make the torte: In the bowl of a stand mixer, place the Swerve, butter, and extract and blend for 8 to 10 minutes until well combined. Scrape down the sides of the bowl as needed.
3. Add the egg yolks and continue to blend until fully combined. Add the almond flour and mix until smooth, then stir in the ricotta and lemon juice.
4. Whisk the egg whites in a separate medium bowl until stiff peaks form. Add the whites to the batter and stir well. Pour the batter into the prepared pan and smooth the top.
5. Place a trivet in the bottom of your Instant Pot and pour in the water. Use a foil sling to lower the baking pan onto the trivet. Tuck in the sides of the sling.
6. Seal the lid, press Pressure Cook or Manual, and set the timer for 30 minutes. Once finished, let the pressure release naturally.
7. Lock the lid. Select the Manual mode and set the cooking time for 30 minutes at High Pressure.
8. When the timer beeps, perform a natural pressure release for 10 minutes. Carefully remove the lid.

9. Use the foil sling to lift the pan out of the Instant Pot. Place the torte in the fridge for 40 minutes to chill before glazing.
10. Meanwhile, make the glaze: Place the butter in a large pan over high heat and cook for about 5 minutes until brown, stirring occasionally. Remove from the heat. While stirring the browned butter, add the Swerve.
11. Carefully add the lemon juice and cream cheese to the butter mixture. Allow the glaze to cool for a few minutes, or until it starts to thicken.
12. Transfer the chilled torte to a serving plate. Pour the glaze over the torte and return it to the fridge to chill for an additional 30 minutes.
13. Scatter the lemon zest on top of the torte and arrange the lemon slices on the plate around the torte.
14. Serve.

Lemon Blueberry Cheesecake

Prep time: 10 minutes | Cook time: 6 minutes | Serves 6

1 tablespoon coconut oil, melted, for greasing the pan

1¼ cups soft pitted Medjool dates, divided

1 cup gluten-free rolled oats

2 cups cashews

1 cup fresh blueberries

3 tablespoons freshly squeezed lemon juice or lime juice

1¾ cups water

Salt, to taste

1. Grease a 6-inch springform pan or pie dish with melted coconut oil.
2. In a food processor, combine 1 cup of dates and the oats. Processor until they form a sticky mixture. Press this mixture into the prepared pan.
3. In a blender, combine the remaining ¼ cup of dates, cashews, blueberries, lemon juice, ¾ cup of water, and a pinch of salt. Blend on high speed for about 1 minute, until smooth and creamy, stopping a couple of times to scrape down the sides. Pour this mixture over the crust. Cover the pan with aluminum foil.
4. Pour the remaining 1 cup of water into the Instant Pot and insert a trivet. Using a foil sling or silicone helper handles, lower the pan onto the trivet.
5. Lock the lid. Select the Manual mode and set the cooking time for 6 minutes at High Pressure.

6. When the timer beeps, perform a natural pressure release for 10 minutes, then release any remaining pressure. Carefully remove the lid.

7. Cool for 5 to 10 minutes before slicing and serving.

Lush Chocolate Cake

Prep time: 10 minutes | Cook time: 35 minutes | Serves 8

For Cake:

2 cups almond flour

⅓ cup unsweetened cocoa powder

1½ teaspoons baking powder

1 cup granulated erythritol

Pinch of salt

4 eggs

1 teaspoon vanilla extract

½ cup butter, melted and cooled

6 tablespoons strong coffee, cooled

½ cup water

For Frosting:

4 ounces (113 g) cream cheese, softened

½ cup butter, softened

¼ teaspoon vanilla extract

2½ tablespoons powdered erythritol

2 tablespoons unsweetened cocoa powder

1. To make the cake: In a large bowl, whisk together the almond flour, cocoa powder, baking powder, granulated erythritol, and salt. Whisk well to remove any lumps.

2. Add the eggs and vanilla and mix with a hand mixer until combined.

3. With the mixer still on low speed, slowly add the melted butter and mix until well combined.

4. Add the coffee and mix on low speed until the batter is thoroughly combined. Scrape the sides and bottom of the bowl to make sure everything is well mixed.

5. Spray the cake pan with cooking spray. Pour the batter into the pan. Cover tightly with aluminum foil.

6. Add the water to the pot. Place the cake pan on the trivet and carefully lower then pan into the pot.

7. Close the lid. Select Manual mode and set cooking time for 35 minutes on High Pressure.

8. When timer beeps, use a quick pressure release and open the lid.

9. Carefully remove the cake pan from the pot and place on a wire rack to cool. Flip the cake onto a plate once it is cool enough to touch. Cool completely before frosting.

10. To make the frosting: In a medium bowl, use the mixer to whip the cream cheese, butter, and vanilla until light and fluffy, 1 to 2 minutes. With the mixer running, slowly add the powdered erythritol and cocoa powder. Mix until everything is well combined.

11. Once the cake is completely cooled, spread the frosting on the top and down the sides.

Tapioca Pudding

Prep time: 12 mins, Cook Time: 15 mins, Servings: 4

- 1 cup water
- 1¼ cups almond milk
- ¼ cup rinsed and drained seed tapioca pearls
- ½ cup sugar
- ½ tsp. lemon zest

1. Pour the water into the Instant Pot.

2. Add the steamer basket inside the pot.

3. In a heat-proof bowl, mix all the ingredients until the sugar has dissolved.

4. Cover with foil and put the bowl on top of the basket.

5. Lock the lid. Set the Instant Pot to Manual mode, then set the timer for 10 minutes at High Pressure.

6. When the timer goes off, perform a natural release for 5 minutes, then release any remaining pressure. Carefully open the lid.

7. Serve immediately or refrigerate for several hours and serve chilled.

Kentucky Butter Cake

Prep time: 5 minutes | Cook time: 35 minutes | Serves 4

2 cups almond flour

¾ cup granulated erythritol

1½ teaspoons baking powder

4 eggs

1 tablespoon vanilla extract

½ cup butter, melted

Cooking spray

½ cup water

1. In a medium bowl, whisk together the almond flour, erythritol, and baking powder. Whisk well to remove any lumps.

2. Add the eggs and vanilla and whisk until combined.

3. Add the butter and whisk until the batter is mostly smooth and well combined.

4. Grease the pan with cooking spray and pour in the batter. Cover tightly with aluminum foil.

5. Add the water to the pot. Place the Bundt pan on the trivet and carefully lower it into the pot using.

6. Set the lid in place. Select the Manual mode and set the cooking time for 35 minutes on High Pressure. When the timer goes off, do a quick pressure release. Carefully open the lid.

7. Remove the pan from the pot. Let the cake cool in the pan before flipping out onto a plate.

Vanilla Crème Brûlée

Prep time: 7 minutes | Cook time: 9 minutes | Serves 4

1 cup heavy cream (or full-fat coconut milk for dairy-free)

2 large egg yolks

2 tablespoons Swerve, or more to taste

Seeds scraped from ½ vanilla bean (about 8 inches long), or 1 teaspoon vanilla extract

1 cup cold water

4 teaspoons Swerve, for topping

1. Heat the cream in a pan over medium-high heat until hot, about 2 minutes.

2. Place the egg yolks, Swerve, and vanilla seeds in a blender and blend until smooth.

3. While the blender is running, slowly pour in the hot cream. Taste and adjust the sweetness to your liking.

4. Scoop the mixture into four ramekins with a spatula. Cover the ramekins with aluminum foil.

5. Add the water to the Instant Pot and insert a trivet. Place the ramekins on the trivet.

6. Lock the lid. Select the Manual mode and set the cooking time for 7 minutes at High Pressure.

7. When the timer beeps, perform a quick pressure release. Carefully remove the lid.

8. Keep the ramekins covered with the foil and place in the refrigerator for about 2 hours until completely chilled.

9. Sprinkle 1 teaspoon of Swerve on top of each crème brûlée. Use the oven broiler to melt the sweetener.

10. Allow the topping to cool in the fridge for 5 minutes before serving.

RECIPE INDEX

Chicken with Jalapeño 50
Chili Chicken Zoodles 54
Chili Endives Platter 118
Chili-Rubbed Tilapia 45
Chinese Flavor Chicken Wings 118
Chinese Steamed Chicken 54
Chipotle Chicken Fajita 54
Chipotle Cilantro Rice 92
Chocolate Almond Fudge 134
Cilantro Lime Rice 93
Cinnamon Brown Rice 93
Cinnamon-Vanilla Applesauce 132
Citrus Beef Carnitas 65
Citrus Buckwheat and Barley Salad 119
Citrus Chicken Tacos 55
Classic Pot Roast 65
Coconut Brown Rice Pudding 136
Coconut Muesli Stuffed Apples 25
Confetti Rice 93
Corn and Mushroom Stock 129
Corned Beef 67
Crack Chicken with Bacon 55
Creamy Chicken with Mushrooms 56
Creamy Tomato Pasta with Spinach 95
Crispy Herbed Chicken 56
Crispy Salmon Fillets 38
Crispy Wings 56
Curried Chicken Legs with Mustard 57
Curried Salmon 41
Curried Sorghum with Golden Raisins 104

D

Daikon and Zucchini Fritters 37
Double-Cheesy Drumsticks 50
Duo-Cheese Mushroom Pasta 98

E

Egg Meatloaf 77
Eggplant Pork Lasagna 77
Eggs En Cocotte 17
Eggs In Purgatory 17

Endives and Lemon Juice Appetizer 120

F

Farro and Cherry Salad 105
Farro Risotto with Mushroom 108
Fennel Chicken 58
Feta and Arugula Pasta Salad 99
Filipino Chicken Adobo 58
Flounder Fillets with Capers 39
French Eggs 18

G

Garlic Chicken 58
Garlicky Baby Bok Choy 30
Garlicky Lamb Leg 84
Garlicky Pork Tenderloin 78
Garlicky Prime Rib 67
Ginger Chicken Congee 59
Ginger Short Ribs 68
Gingered Beef Tenderloin 68
Ginger-Garlic Spicy Kale 126
Golden Bacon Sticks 78
Greek Beef and Spinach Ravioli 68
Greek Lamb Leg 84
Greek Lamb Loaf 84
Greek Quinoa Bowl 105
Greek Snapper 46
Green Beans with Toasted Peanuts 29
Green Tea Risotto 95
Ground Beef Pasta 95

H

Halibut En Papillote 40
Halibut Stew with Bacon 40
Hard-Boiled Eggs 24
Harissa Lamb 85
Hawaiian Pulled Pork Roast with Cabbage 78
Hawaiian Sweet Potato Hash 19
Herbed Beef Chuck Roast 72
Herbed Cod Steaks 41
Herbed Lamb Shank 85
Herbed Red Snapper 46

Herbed Sirloin Tip Roast 69
Honey Carrot Salad 30
Honey-Glazed Chicken with Sesame 59
Huli Huli Chicken 59

I

Icelandic Lamb with Turnip 85
Indian Butter Chicken 59
Indian Lamb Curry 85
Indian Lamb Korma 86
Indian Roasted Pork 79
Indian Spicy Beef with Basmati 70
Instant Pot Jasmine Rice 96
Instant Pot Ranch Chicken 60
Instant Pot Rib 79
Instant Pot Rib Roast 70
Italian Carrot and Potato Medley 32
Italian Pork Cutlets 79
Italian Salmon with Lemon Juice 41

J

Jalapeño Peanuts 120
Jamaican Curry Chicken Drumsticks 60
Jamaican Pork Roast 80
Japanese Beef Shanks 67
Jollof Rice 96

K

Kentucky Butter Cake 141
Keto Brownies 139
Khoreshe Karafs 30
Kidney Bean Stew 112
Kimchi Pasta 94
Korean Beef Ribs 71
Kung Pao Chicken 57

L

Lamb and Tomato Bhuna 87
Lamb Burgers 84
Lamb Casserole 89
Lamb Curry 83
Lamb Curry with Tomatoes 87

Lamb Meatballs 86
Lamb Rogan Josh 89
Lamb with Anchovies 88
Leek and Asparagus Frittata 21
Lemon and Ricotta Torte 140
Lemon Beef Meal 71
Lemon Blueberry Cheesecake 140
Lemon Pepper Salmon 42
Lemongrass Rice and Beef Pot 71
Lemony Salmon with Avocados 42
Lentil Soup with Garam Masala 112
Lentils with Spinach 107
Lettuce Wrapped Chicken Sandwich 20
Lime Tilapia Fillets 43
Lime-Chili Chicken 54
Little Smokies with Grape Jelly 121
Lush Chocolate Cake 141
Lush Veg Medley 32

M

Maple Syrup Lemon Pudding 139
Maple-Glazed Spareribs 80
Marinara Sauce 129
Marsala Tofu Pasta 94
Mediterranean Couscous Salad 107
Mexican Beef Shred 72
Mexican Chili Pork 80
Mexican Rice 98
Millet and Brown Lentil Chili 113
Mini Bell Pepper and Cheddar Frittata 21
Moong Bean with Cabbage 107
Mujadara (Lebanese Lentils and Rice) 108
Mushroom Alfredo Rice 94
Mushroom Barley Risotto 108
Mushroom Beef Stroganoff 69
Mushroom Broth 130
Mushrooms with Garlic 31
Mussel Appetizer 119
Mustard Macaroni and Cheese 99

O

Oat and Black Bean Brownies 135
Orange and Strawberry Compote 25
Osso Buco with Gremolata 66

P

Panko Tilapia 43
Paprika Chicken with Tomatoes 60
Paprika Pork with Brussels Sprouts 81
Parmesan Drumsticks 61
Parmesan Pea Risotto 97
Pasta Carbonara 96
Pecan and Cherry Stuffed Pumpkin 29
Penne Pasta with Tomato-Vodka Sauce 100
Pepper and Egg Oatmeal Bowl 105
Perch Fillets with Red Curry 43
Pesto Fish Packets with Parmesan 39
Pesto Halibut 40
Pesto Salmon with Almonds 44
Pesto Spaghetti Squash 125
Pizza Pasta 91
Pork and Beef Chili Nachos 118
Pork and Carrot Broth 130
Pork and Mushroom with Mustard 81
Pork Quill Egg Cups 22
Pork Shoulder and Celery 82
Pork Steaks with Pico de Gallo 77
Pork with Bell Peppers 81
Pork with Brussels Sprouts 82
Potato Cubes 120
Prosciutto-Wrapped Chicken 61
Pulled Pork 81
Pumpkin Oatmeal 23

Q

Quick Salmon 44
Quinoa and Bean Chili 114

R

Raisin, Apple, and Pecan Oatmeal 21
Ranch Dip 130
Ratatouille 126
Ratatouille 31

Red Curry Halibut 44
Rhubarb Compote 23
Ritzy Green Pea and Cauliflower Curry 33
Roasted Lamb Leg 87

S

Salmon Cakes 44
Salmon Head Soup 115
Salmon Packets 38
Salmon Stew 115
Salmon with Basil Pesto 45
Salmon with Broccoli 39
Salmon with Dijon Mustard 38
Salmon with Dill 45
Salmon with Honey Sauce 41
Salmon with Lemon Mustard 47
Salmon with Mayo 43
Salsa Chicken Legs 61
Satarash with Eggs 33
Satay Sauce 130
Sautéed Beef and Green Beans 72
Sautéed Brussels Sprouts And Pecans 33
Seafood Stock 131
Sesame Bok Choy 34
Sesame Chicken 62
Shredded Chicken 62
Shrimp and Tomatoes 117
Simple Chocolate Cake 138
Simple Instant Pot Pearl Barley 104
Simple Wild Brown Rice 98
Sirloin with Snap Peas 69
Sloppy Joes 66
Slow Cooked Beef Pizza Casserole 72
Slow Cooked Beef Steak 73
Slow Cooked Lamb Shanks 88
Smoky Chicken 62
Snapper with Spicy Tomato Sauce 45
Spaghetti Squash Noodles 34
Spaghetti Squash Noodles with Tomatoes 34
Spaghetti Squash with Olives 125
Spaghetti Squash with Spinach 28

Special White Pancake 24
Spiced Chicken Drumsticks 62
Spiced Fruit Medley 23
Spiced Orange Carrots 126
Spicy Chicken with Smoked Sausage 63
Spicy Green Beans 126
Spicy Lamb Shoulder 88
Spicy Minced Lamb Meat 89
Spinach and Feta Stuffed Chicken 63
Spinach and Ham Frittata 19
Spinach and Mushroom Pasta 99
Spinach and Pine Nut Fusilli Pasta 95
Spinach and Tomato Couscous 109
Spinach Lemon Pasta 97
Spinach with Almonds and Olives 35
Sriracha Collard Greens 127
Steak and Bell Pepper Fajitas 73
Steak, Pepper, and Lettuce Salad 73
Steamed Artichoke with Aioli Sauce 127
Steamed Asparagus 31
Steamed Asparagus with Mustard Dip 121
Steamed Cod and Veggies 46
Steamed Salmon 39
Steel-Cut Oatmeal 21
Stone Fruit Compote 24
Strawberry and Pumpkin Spice Quinoa Bowl 25
Stuffed Eggs 121
Summer Chili 114
Sumptuous Beef and Tomato Biryani 74
Sumptuous Navy Beans 109
Super Bean and Grain Burgers 110
Super Beef Chili 74
Super Chocolate Cookies 138
Super Garlicky Chicken 53
Sweet Apricot Beef 74
Sweet Potato and Kale Egg Bites 25
Sweet Potato Beef 75
Sweet Roasted Cashews 122
Sweet-and-Sour Kale and Beets 125

T

Tabasco Sauce 131
Tapioca Pudding 141
Tequila Short Ribs 75
Teriyaki Salmon 47
Tex Mex Tofu Scramble 26
Thai Coconut Beef with Snap Peas 75
Thai Fish Curry 47
Thai Peanut Chicken 64
Thousand Island Dressing 131
Three Bean Salad with Parsley 122
Thyme Carrots 122
Thyme Chicken with Brussels Sprouts 64
Thyme-Sesame Crusted Halibut 47
Tilapia Fillets with Arugula 42
Tilapia Fish Cakes 47
Tilapia with Pineapple Salsa 48
Tofu and Kale Miso Soup 112
Tofu and Mango Curry 35
Tomatillo and Jackfruit Tinga 32
Tomato and Chickpea Rice 92
Tomato and Parsley Quinoa Salad 122
Tomato Salsa 132
Tropical Fruit Chutney 26
Tuna Fillets with Lemon Butter 48
Tuna Noodle Casserole 48
Tuna Noodle Casserole with Cheese 101
Tuna Salad with Lettuce 49
Tuna with Eggs 38
Turkey Spaghetti 91

V

Vanilla Applesauce 26
Vanilla Crème Brûlée 142
Vanilla Pancake 18
Vanilla Rice Pudding 123
Vegan Rice Pudding 101
Vegetable Basmati Rice 101
Vegetable Biryani 104
Vegetable Chicken Skewers 117
Vegetable Fried Millet 110
Vegetable Pasta 101

Vegetable Quinoa Stew 112
Vegetable Stock 132
Vegetarian Mac and Cheese 36
Vegetarian Smothered Cajun Greens 36
Vegetarian Thai Pineapple Fried Rice 102
Veggie Quiche 27
Veggie Stew 31
Vinegary Broccoli with Cheese 36
Vinegary Brown Rice Noodles 102
Vinegary Pearl Onion 123
Vinegary Pork Chops with Figs and Pears 82

W

Walnut and Pear Oatmeal 22
Watercress Appetizer Salad 123
Western Omelet 27
Wheat Berry and Celery Salad 116
White Beans with Poblano and Tomatillos 111

Whole Roasted Chicken with Lemon and Rosemary 64
Wild Alaskan Cod with Cherry Tomatoes 49
Wild Rice and Basmati Pilaf 102
Wild Rice and Kale Salad 120
Winter Beef Roast Pot 76
Winter Chili 115

Z

Za'atar-Spiced Bulgur Wheat Salad 111
Zoodles with Mediterranean Sauce 36
Zucchini and Bell Pepper Stir Fry 37
Zucchini and Chickpea Tagine 128
Zucchini and Tomato Melange 37
Zucchini Penne Pasta 100
Zucchini Spread 123
Zucchini Sticks 31
Zucchini-Parmesan Cheese Fritters 128

CPSIA information can be obtained
at www.ICGtesting.com
Printed in the USA
BVHW011042180621
609824BV00008B/1870

9 781914 923036